Professor Kerryn Phelps AM is a docto
rights advocate, past president of the Au
past president Australasian Integrative Me
Professor in the Faculty of Medicine at
Wales and Adjunct Professor at Sydney Medical
of Sydney. She is co-author of a textbook *General Practice: The Integrative Approach* and mother of three. She is the founder and medical director of Cooper Street Clinic general practice and uclinic integrative medicine clinic in Sydney Australia. In 2003 she was awarded the Centenary Medal for services to Health and Medicine and in 2011 she was named a Member of the Order of Australia for service to medicine, particularly through leadership roles with the Australian Medical Association, education and community health, and as a general practitioner. She lives in Sydney with her wife, Jackie, daughter, Gabi, and their toy poodles Paris and Lulu. To find out more visit www.drkerrynphelps.com.

ULTIMATE WELLNESS

The 3-step plan

PROFESSOR KERRYN PHELPS AM

MACMILLAN
Pan Macmillan Australia

First published 2013 in Macmillan by Pan Macmillan Australia Pty Limited
1 Market Street, Sydney

National Library of Australia
Cataloguing-in-Publication data:

Phelps, Kerryn.
Prof. Kerryn Phelps' ultimate wellness : the 3-step plan /
Prof. Kerryn Phelps.
9781742611921 (pbk.)
Health. Medical care. Lifestyles.
613

Case histories included in this book are de-identified and fictionalised compilations of
representative cases for the purposes of illustration only. Any resemblance to persons
living or dead is purely coincidental.

Text design by Studio Emma
Typeset in Adobe Caslon Pro by Midland Typesetters, Australia
Printed in Australia by McPherson's Printing Group

Papers used by Pan Macmillan Australia Pty Ltd are natural, recyclable products made
from wood grown in sustainable forests. The manufacturing processes conform to the
environmental regulations of the country of origin.

The publishers and their respective employers or agents will not accept responsibility for
any injury or damage to any person as a result of participation in the activities described
by this book.

For Jackie ... just because!

Table of Contents

MY JOURNEY: PART ONE

Back in 2003, I was just a few months away from finishing my term as President of the Australian Medical Association. It had been three years lived at a cracking pace. I had been working ridiculously long hours, sometimes up to 18 hours a day; traversing the continent, living between Sydney, Canberra and whatever other destination I was visiting that week; and trying to run my practice and manage my family responsibilities. I was walking most days, but getting nowhere near the level of exercise I had done previously or the amount I knew I needed to do to keep my fitness up. With all of the travel and meetings running through mealtimes, an ideal diet was elusive and I had put on a few kilos. To say the medico-political environment I was working in was stressful is an understatement.

I was in my early forties at the time and I noticed my cycle became erratic. Big surprise! I put it down to stress but didn't take the time to look at the underlying cause of the problem because I was so distracted by the intensity of the work I was doing, and I guess subconsciously I thought I could put my wellbeing on the backburner until the job was done. I now know this was an excuse, not a reason.

I spoke to my gynaecologist who prescribed a hormone treatment. I also had a bad cold with a cough, but when the cold cleared, the cough just wouldn't go away. Then a few weeks later I noticed I was having trouble walking up hills. I made a mental note that I was letting myself get unfit and I needed to pay attention to my exercise program once my cough got better.

Then the next day I couldn't get up the stairs without stopping because I was short of breath.

The day after that was a particularly busy day. I was working at my clinic in the morning, then I was delivering a lecture on medical indemnity reform to law students at the University of New South Wales, then dashing to the airport for a crucial meeting in Canberra with then prime minister John Howard. In the evening I had a full schedule too: a massive pile of paperwork, a meeting with my AMA colleagues and a political dinner to attend.

But by then I couldn't make it across the consulting room without losing my breath. I knew something was seriously wrong.

I called the professor of respiratory medicine at St Vincent's Hospital in Sydney. He insisted I come straight in. I remember deliberating about whether I could fit it into my terribly busy schedule but I decided I should go.

Later I would be told that if I had tried to get on that plane to Canberra, I would likely not have survived to tell you this story, or to write this book. Even making it to hospital, I had just over 10 per cent chance of surviving, less of surviving without disability.

Within an hour of arriving at the hospital, I was in intensive care with a confirmed, life-threatening pulmonary embolism, an adverse effect from the hormone treatment I had started taking just weeks before. Blood clots were filling about half of both of my lungs. I was on oxygen, had monitors across my chest and was being injected with blood thinning medication. The next few days were a blur of blood tests, CT scans and ultrasounds.

We could clear the clots with anticoagulant injections but for a full recovery, the treatment required a broader view. I was facing a health crisis with serious ongoing consequences. It was a fork in the road. What was I going to do? How could I make changes to my life to find perspective, look after the fundamentals like exercise, diet, sleep and stress management? How could I overcome the fatigue and recover my fitness? How could I fit the exercise I knew I had to do into the frantically busy life I was leading? And how could I plan my later years knowing that hormone replacement was off the agenda if menopause struck with a vengeance?

It was time for a reality check.

My 'brush with death' forced me to face life with a new perspective.

It also forced me to face anew my attitudes to the practice of medicine and the choices we can offer for real and effective health improvement. And yes, to believe that every person can set themselves on the path to ultimate wellness.

My treating physician spoke to me before I left hospital to rehabilitate. He was absolutely unambiguous about two things: continuing the anti-coagulant injections for a few months to dissolve the clots; and I had to exercise for an hour every day to maintain my cardio vascular fitness. *No excuses*. I might have lots of reasons why it might be difficult,: 'Not enough time', 'too busy', 'I have to fly interstate', 'I have to finish writing a speech' – but none of them were good enough. There really was no excuse good enough for not making the changes that would aid my recovery from this life-threatening illness and optimise my wellbeing into the future.

I got to about 80 out of 100 on my personal scale of wellness but that was not going to be good enough. My recovery was a long road. I'll tell you more about it later. But I made it. You can too.

I can honestly say every time I go for a walk on the beach or a swim or a long paddle in the kayak or ski down a mountain, I say a quiet word of gratitude for being able to do it. I am fitter and stronger than ever.

This book is my way of sharing what I have learned from my decades in medical practice, as well as an epiphany or two from my own personal journey. I overhauled my health and changed my life for the better. I found my own new normal and now, with my help, I hope you can too.

WHY ULTIMATE WELLNESS?

Are you fatigued? Stressed? Irritable? Sluggish? Are you prone to lots of annoying minor illnesses?

Are you trying to get your mojo back after a debilitating illness? Or do you just feel 'pretty ordinary'? Maybe you have been to your doctor and were told they can't find anything wrong with you. But still you know that things are just not right.

In medical practice, and in the health system generally, we spend most of our time diagnosing and treating people with major illnesses or significant threats to their health. Some of the patients I see are seriously ill, and are faced with the challenge of trying to survive. Others are recovering from illness or surgery the best they can. Traditionally, most medical treatment is about the aim of getting patients from poor health or life-threatening circumstances to a 'cure' or, where that is impossible, to a state of well-controlled chronic disease management.

If ultimate wellness is 100 on a scale of one to 100, you could say we are trying to get people from somewhere above zero to about 50 to 80. But there is this whole other group of people who don't have an actual disease that we can slap a label on but they just don't feel 100 per cent.

When it comes to managing illness or planning health goals, I find many people set their personal wellness bar way too low. They settle for feeling just okay, when they could feel so much better. So many people don't even know they are not as well as they could be. You may have no idea how much better you have the capacity to feel because it has been so long, if ever, since you have experienced truly optimal health.

So, what about this concept of getting you from ranking an average 50 to 80 on our scale of wellness, up closer to that ultimate level of 100? How could you possibly achieve this?

You may already know a lot of the information in this book. In which case, the trick is to find the motivation to put your knowledge into action – and we'll talk about that too. A great deal of what you need to do to achieve optimal health is actually dependent upon you swapping old, unhealthy patterns for new, healthier ones, and then feeling the difference.

Health is not just about an overloaded system of hospitals and nurses or doctors to do procedures or provide therapies to sick people; so much of your wellbeing is about the individual decisions and choices you make every hour of every day. Many of those decisions lead you down the path to feeling under par, and many of them will, over time, eventually accumulate to create overt disease. I will show you how to counteract the enemies of good health: stress, poor diet, lack of sleep, lack of exercise and unhealthy or even dangerous lifestyle habits. Knowledge and the motivation to apply that knowledge are the fuel. The fuel to be the best you can be, to feel truly vibrant and energetic.

Every day I see people who neglect the basics, such as nutrition, life management, healthy habits, health check-ups or exercise. They wait until a health disaster happens, then go out and spend a fortune on treatments that don't necessarily work.

In recent times there has been a vigorous and at times bitter debate about the scientific evidence base of some of the so-called complementary therapies. There is an equally bitter debate about the risks of conventional medical treatments when less harmful lifestyle changes or non-medical therapies may get you equivalent or better results without the risk of serious adverse events. My aim is to help you navigate through some of the claims and counter-claims about which activities, actions, treatments or practitioners might or might not be helpful to you. I will also tell you how to safely combine therapies so that you can benefit from a range of healthcare interventions.

Many medical and other health practitioners treat only one little bit of you or one part of the problem, rather than the whole of you and all the things that impact on your health. This book is about helping you to find the right practitioner for the right problem, and what you can do for yourself to optimise your own wellbeing.

Ultimate Wellness: The 3-Step Plan will show you how, in the three stages of AUDIT, REBOOT and SUSTAIN, you can experience a personal transformation.

Ultimate Wellness: The 3-Step Plan is about taking control of your health, helping you to protect your health, working out what actions you need to take and showing you how to access the best sort of treatment if and when you need it.

This book is also about showing you how to help yourself by engaging with the basics of good health as well as how to achieve ultimate wellness through the sensible and wise use of conventional and complementary therapies.

Once you know there can be a healthier, more energetic version of yourself, make the decision to take action. The time is now!

THINKING OUTSIDE THE SQUARE

As children, we grow up with a family folklore that coalesces from the stories we hear across generations, and the experiences we share. Although I am the first doctor in my extended family – in fact, I was the first in my family to have a university degree – I am not the first 'healer'.

Everyone spoke of my grandmother as having 'healing hands' because of her extraordinary sense of what to do when one of her brood had an illness or injury. One of many children, she grew up in an era when pharmaceutical drugs had not yet been developed, and communities had to rely on traditional healing practices and hoping for the power of the body to heal itself. Recipes for poultices and potions were handed down from one generation to the next, and those with the knowledge shared their skills for the benefit of those who could not afford to visit a doctor.

One story that looms large in our family history happened to my grandfather during World War II. Following the Great Depression, he had gone to Papua New Guinea to work in the goldfields and was caught up in the Japanese invasion. Isolated and left to fend for themselves, he and several other mine-workers had just one option: to walk out of the treacherous jungle of the Owen Stanley Ranges.

Back home, my grandfather's wife and children had been told he was missing, believed killed. Over many months, the men made their way on foot to the coast, and then by canoe across the Coral Sea to northern Australia. By the time he arrived back on home soil, he was unrecognisable. He had lost half his body weight, was suffering crippling fevers from malaria, and had an infection so serious that doctors at the hospital declared they were planning to amputate his foot.

'Not on your life,' said my grandmother. She took him home and set to work with her poultices and potions, and a large dose of good old home cooking. Yes, she saved his foot, and he recovered to live to 86 years. His recovery would have been much faster if, along with my grandmother's healing practices, he had had access to the medications we now take for granted, such as antibiotics. Now, of course, we have many options.

Fast-forward to my own childhood, where my parents strongly emphasised a sporty outdoor lifestyle, fresh food and loads of time spent in natural environments observing the phenomena of the seasons and tides. I think the only time I saw a doctor was to get patched up after an accident while rockclimbing or sailing or playing hockey.

When I had my own children, instinct and medical training drove me to make sure I raised them with as healthy an environment and lifestyle as possible. As a result of that healthy start and fortuitous genes, both my adult children are robust and rarely sick. They also both work in health care, my daughter as a dietitian and my son as an aged-care nurse. My youngest daughter is growing up with a strong sense that she can have control over her wellbeing through the decisions she makes.

So my philosophy of health and wellbeing, which I bring to this book, is drawn from a family history of natural and traditional healing practices, an appreciation of the environment, a highly disciplined and scientific medical school and hospital-trained background, and over 30 years of clinical experience solving a multitude of simple and complex health problems.

THE APPROACH OF THIS BOOK

Ultimate Wellness: The 3-Step Plan will guide you through a process where you will:

- *AUDIT your life and lifestyle,*
- *REBOOT your life habits and attitudes, then*
- *SUSTAIN the changes that will benefit your wellbeing throughout your life, without feeling as though you are missing out, and transition into a new healthy lifestyle that will become your 'new normal'.*

HEALTH CARE APPROACHES

You will often see the broad therapeutic approaches within health care described as 'traditional' or 'conventional' medicine, 'orthodox' or 'unorthodox' medicine, 'holistic' or 'integrative' or 'complementary and alternative' medicine (known by the acronym CAM). These are just artificial demarcations for a number of reasons. There have been many attempts at defining CAM and a frequently cited definition is:

... a broad domain of healing resources that encompasses all health systems, modalities, and practices and their accompanying theories and beliefs, other than those intrinsic to the politically dominant health system of a particular society or culture in a given historical period.
(INSTITUTE OF MEDICINE 2005).

What is considered alternative in one culture might be considered completely conventional or mainstream in another culture. And even within a culture, there is increasingly a crossover in what is accepted as a conventional treatment, depending on its level of acceptance by the dominant medical fraternity at any given point in history, and what is considered complementary or alternative. For example, early in my career, acupuncture was considered an unorthodox or alternative practice in Western medicine. These days, a significant proportion of doctors have trained in acupuncture and use it in their daily practice, while an even greater number refer patients for acupuncture treatment, placing it in the conventional or orthodox category. Of course, if you happen to live in China, acupuncture has been a part of the predominant medical culture for thousands of years.

Over my years in primary care, I have become increasingly intrigued by a philosophy of health care called 'integrative medicine'. This awareness arose out of a gradual realisation that while my conventional Western medical training was a brilliant basis for medical practice, it did not come close to providing the answers to all of the problems I would be asked to solve in clinical practice. I needed to cast my net wider. Beyond thinking outside the square, I had to think as though there was no square.

DEFINITION OF INTEGRATIVE MEDICINE

Integrative medicine (IM) is the practice of medicine that reaffirms the importance of the relationship between practitioner and patient, focuses on the whole person, is informed by evidence, and makes use of all appropriate therapeutic approaches, healthcare professionals and disciplines to achieve optimal health and healing.

DEVELOPED AND ADOPTED BY THE CONSORTIUM, MAY 2004
EDITED MAY 2005, MAY 2009 AND NOVEMBER 2009

Integrative medicine is the practice of medicine that aims to incorporate the best, most appropriate and safest types of treatment, regardless of their original source. IM is grounded in conventional medicine, particularly in the emphasis on accurate diagnosis and having a scientific basis for treatment decisions. Lifestyle advice and evidence-based complementary medicine are also prescribed and may be used as a range of possible options, either instead of standard medical treatment or, more commonly, in addition to it. Consider the example of someone with heart disease. They need the highly technical medical treatment and medications to save their life in the event of a heart attack, but IM will also incorporate other elements such as a detailed exercise program; changes in their diet; the prescribing of appropriate vitamins, minerals, herbs and other supplements; and stress management techniques such as meditation. The aim of this book is to guide you in devising your own 'best practice'.

The medical consultation of today is vastly different from 20 or 30 years ago. Nowadays, it is more of a bilateral discussion, sometimes a negotiation about what treatment feels right to the patient at that particular time. Through public health initiatives, health promotion through the media and, of course, the rise of the internet, non-medical people now have the ability to get hold of accurate and credible medical information and understand it and use it to make appropriate health decisions. This is what we call 'health literacy'.

The US Department of Health and Human Services defines health literacy as: 'The degree to which individuals have the capacity to obtain, process and understand basic health information and services needed to make appropriate health decisions'. This definition acknowledges the fact that health literacy operates within 'the complex group of reading, listening, analytical and decision making skills' and is dependent upon 'the ability to apply these skills to health situations'.

Functional literacy refers to what literacy enables you to do with that information.

From the perspective of a GP, I see some huge advantages with this new style of consultative practice.

I like to redefine medical treatment, because a lot of the treatment I prescribe is about lifestyle changes. This might involve advice about stopping smoking, taking up exercise or changing a dietary pattern. For this type of treatment to have a chance of success, a patient has to understand why it is important, and then have the motivation to make the changes and be prepared to sustain them. The same goes for any medical advice or prescription. Unless there is an understanding of the reason for the advice or prescription as well as that essential ingredient – the motivation to follow the advice – then it just won't happen.

So with health literacy comes the move towards self-management of health care. This means that you as the patient or consumer are in the driving seat as far as your healthcare decisions are concerned. Your medical and health care advisers perform various functions with your consent. This might be an investigation, a blood test, a surgical procedure, a prescription for a course of medication, the formulation of a plan for cancer treatment or a recommendation for a lifestyle intervention.

Self-management does not mean having to be your own doctor.

> Rather than simply 'self-management', I prefer to call it 'guided self-management'.

SELF-PRESCRIBING

Self-prescribing or self-medication is a part of this spectrum of self-management and is usually described as the use of substances, including medications, supplements, alcohol and comfort food, to maintain wellbeing, relieve symptoms or manage health problems. Many people have one or more general practitioners and, if necessary, their medical specialist(s) they see, hopefully on a regular basis for medical check-ups and management of health problems. In addition, most people see other types of practitioners or advisers. They probably see a combination of several practitioners at different times.

You might have been prescribed medicines, therapies, herbs and supplements by a professional, and you might also have added in things you buy over the counter, which you have read about in a magazine or on the internet, or you have been told about by a friend. If this sounds like you, the dangers are obvious.

People who want to use alternative therapies but use them badly or poorly, or mix them up with pharmaceutical or conventional medical treatments without good knowledge place themselves at risk of serious consequences. There are two dangers with a higgledy-piggledy concoction of therapies. First, you may not be getting the greatest health benefit from an uncoordinated approach – you could be wasting time and money, not getting the 'best bang for your buck' as they say. More seriously, the combinations or doses of substances you are taking might cancel each other out, or be dangerous or ineffective in combination with each other.

What I am proposing here is a well-informed, well-documented, guided and supervised, sensible wellness plan. It is a plan based on consultation with your GP and other trained health professionals, informing yourself, working out what you want to change and why, and then making the changes you decide are important to achieving ultimate wellness.

MOTIVATION AND CHANGE

For successful guided self-management, you need to understand what motivates you.

Maybe you want to take responsibility for maintaining or improving your wellbeing, or you want to have control over health decisions that will affect you.

Some people I see are worried because they have had a problem with prescribed treatment or do not trust advice they have been given in the past and want to know what they can safely do to manage a health problem while minimising medication. I also see a lot of people who have waited until disaster struck before they thought about getting a regular doctor or starting to have proper check-ups.

You could say, 'Oh well, it's never too late,' but in the life and death world of medicine, sometimes it really is too late. Sometimes people come to the realisation that smoking really is bad for them after they find out they have an inoperable lung cancer with a prognosis of less than six months.

Some cancers, like pancreatic cancer, are unpredictable and, as the situation currently stands, unpreventable. Others, such as bowel cancer and cervical cancer, are almost entirely preventable. From the point of view of the patient or their family, dealing with a bowel cancer that has spread to a point where it results in their certain death is a personal tragedy. But from a doctor's point of view, it is also devastating because we know that with early detection and intervention it can be prevented or cured. All it takes is regular check-ups and meticulous follow-up. The majority of skin cancers can also be successfully treated and cured in the early stages.

You can prevent many chronic diseases if you notice the early warning signs and act upon them in their early stages before damage is irreversible or irreparable.

To have a real and sustainable impact on your ultimate wellbeing, you need to ask yourself some serious questions about what you:

- *need to change*
- *want to change*
- *are prepared to do to manifest change*
- *are willing to continue as a long-term sustainable lifestyle in order to achieve your long-term goals.*

GUIDED OR NEGOTIATED SELF-MANAGEMENT PLAN

❧ FIRST GET THE DIAGNOSIS RIGHT

To safely and efficiently manage your own health you need knowledge, good advice and motivation. But you also need a correct diagnosis. For example, there is no point planning to solve your problem of fatigue until you rule out causes like iron deficiency, anaemia, a chronic gut infection, gluten intolerance, an underactive thyroid or one of the other myriad of possible causes for fatigue.

Please don't try to work out the cause of your symptoms yourself. Diagnostic skill is a more complicated art than it might appear. At worst, you will miss something significant, or worry yourself sick thinking you have something serious when actually you do not. By all means work with your doctor to discover or eliminate potential diagnoses, but I strongly advise you not to rely on self-diagnosis and self-prescribing, because it can delay you getting the correct diagnosis and treatment, or set you on the wrong track.

To achieve this will mean gathering a team of health professionals you like and trust to help guide you, starting with a good GP. (See the chapter 'Choosing the Right Health Professionals' on page 34.)

❧ THINK ABOUT ADVERSE EVENTS AND SAFETY

When you embark on a new health routine, it is important to fully inform yourself. If there is even the slightest potential for health or safety concerns related to any intervention you might be planning, it is always wise to seek appropriate counsel.

One suggestion I have is for you to think of a hierarchy of caution related to potential risks from 'likely to be completely safe' on a scale up to 'likely to cause significant adverse effects' in the short or long term. For example, you would not need to be too worried about aromatherapy or gentle exercise, so they would be low on your hierarchy of caution. You would be wise to ask for more information about anything you swallow, anything that breaches the skin (such as acupuncture) or any manipulative therapies (such as osteopathy) because they would deserve a higher degree of caution on the scale.

You need to know the possible risks, precautions and contraindications of any substance you want to take, whether that is a pharmaceutical or 'natural' supplement. I strongly advise you to read any available official Consumer Medicines Information leaflet provided with any therapeutic products or ask for professional advice. Your doctor, pharmacist or other health professional can talk to you about what the potential benefits and risks might be for you.

An intervention or activity can also have adverse effects such as injury. Before you consent to an intervention, ask questions. Procedures such as chemotherapy, radiotherapy, surgery or other medical interventions require the highest degree of caution and information on the potential risks versus the potential benefits.

❧ YOUR PLAN FOR ULTIMATE WELLNESS

As you journey through the book, I will guide you along the process of setting your goals and developing your personal plan to achieve ultimate wellness. Here, briefly, are the steps you will take.

Audit

- *Audit your lifestyle factors and health behaviours and assess what you need to change. Set up an information and symptoms diary. This will be where you make notes about what you eat, what you drink, what exercise you do, how you are sleeping, how you are feeling.*
- *As part of this stage, I advise you to see your doctor for an accurate medical diagnosis to establish your health status, including working out if you have any underlying cause for your health problems that needs to be corrected.*

Reboot

- *Once you have audited your lifestyle, you will figure out what you want to change.*
- *Work out what other advice or treatment you may need to seek.*
- *Assess your capacity and willingness to self-manage part or all of the process.*
- *Develop a symptom management action plan.*
- *Arrange regular preventive health check-ups.*
- *Make a plan for ongoing support, including a regular team of appropriate healthcare professionals.*
- *Assess the lines of communication between you and health practitioners and between your healthcare professionals.*
- *Obtain copies of written information; check recommended websites.*

Sustain

- *Once you have completed the audit and reboot phases, the challenge will be to work out how to successfully sustain the program by incorporating wellbeing practices into your life because you WANT to maintain your newly discovered sense of ultimate wellbeing as your 'new normal'.*

- *We'll look at each of these steps in detail throughout the book, beginning with the first step: your comprehensive Health Audit. Ready when you are!*

Step 1

AUDIT

Health Audit

INTRODUCTION

For a health audit to be useful to you, it has to be honest. Completing an audit is an opportunity to look carefully into the areas of your health that are going as well as possible, and identifying the areas where you need to focus your attention and make changes.

The way to get the best result from your audit is to think long and hard about the answers before you give them and really be as accurate as you can. While it is important to take a careful look at all aspects of your health and health behaviour, you will probably want to prioritise your main problem areas or health concerns. Your opinion is the one that matters most here, but you might engage your partner, friends or health professionals for their perspectives on areas that need attention.

This is a private audit and is not intended as a judgement, other than it will help you judge for yourself any areas you can improve. You can use this audit as a guide to which parts of the book to visit first, or to start a discussion with your doctor or healthcare advisers. Material from the audit is also available at www.drkerrynphelps.com.

HEALTH AUDIT

ENERGY

Rate your energy level on a scale of 1 to 5, 1 being very low energy, 5 being peak energy

	1	2	3	4	5
On waking					
Around midday					
Mid afternoon					
In the evening					

The value of this self-assessment is a good overall indicator. It will give you and your health advisers a guide to the reasons you might be experiencing low energy at certain times of the day. That might relate to sleep patterns, diet, work situation or other factors. It also gives you a comparison to assess your progress as you make changes.

WHAT ARE YOUR MAIN HEALTH CONCERNS RIGHT NOW?

1. _____
2. _____
3. _____
4. _____
5. _____

WHAT MEDICAL PROBLEMS HAVE YOU BEEN DIAGNOSED WITH?

YEAR	DIAGNOSIS/TREATMENT/OUTCOME

HEALTH CARE

Have you had any admissions to hospital in the past five years?

_____

Why?

_____

WHO ARE THE HEALTHCARE PROFESSIONALS YOU HAVE CONSULTED IN THE PAST TWO YEARS?

DO YOU HAVE COPIES OF THEIR REPORTS, OPINIONS OR ADVICE?

Practitioner	Discipline/speciality/ reason	Satisfaction with outcome?

WHAT INVESTIGATIONS HAVE YOU HAD?

Test	Type	Who ordered it?	Result
Blood tests			
X-rays			
CT scans			
MRI			
Ultrasounds			
Special investigations (e.g. colonoscopy, mammogram)			

Obtain and file copies of results in chronological order

WHEN WAS YOUR LAST MEDICAL CHECK-UP?

Within the past year _____

Between 1 and 3 years ago _____

More than 3 years ago _____

   Refer to the chapter 'Choosing the Right Health Professionals' on page 34.

WHEN WAS YOUR LAST DENTAL CHECKUP?

Within 12 months _____
Over 12 months _____
Recommended: a dental checkup every six months.

HOW DO YOU MEASURE UP?

Height H (in metres) _____
Weight W (in kilograms) _____
Body Mass Index (BMI) W(kg)/H(m) × H(m) (This calculation can be confusing. There are online tools that can calculate it for you. What you do is take your weight in kilos and divide it by your height in metres. Then divide that number by your height in metres.) _____
Depending on this number – your BMI – you will get an indication of how your body weight relates to your health risk.
Ideal BMI: 18.5–25
Too light: less than 18.5
Overweight: more than 25
Obese: more than 30

❧ WAIST MEASUREMENT

Hold a tape measure against your skin and breathe out normally. Measure around your waist halfway between your lowest rib and the top of your hipbone, roughly in line with your belly button.
Waist measurement (centimetres) _____
Increased risk:
Men: more than 94 cm
Women: more than 80 cm
Greatly increased risk:
Men: more than 102 cm
Women: more than 88 cm
Refer to the chapters 'Nutrition' on page 132 and 'Exercise' on page 171.

SLEEP

A sleep diary will show you sleep behaviours and patterns that will help ascertain whether sleep is a problem for you, and act as a guide to solve sleep problems. See the table below for an example.

	MON	TUES	WED	THUR	FRI	SAT	SUN
What time did you go to bed?							
Time you spent reading/watching TV in bed before sleep?							
Time taken to go to sleep?							
How many times did you wake in the night? At what times? Why?							
How many hours did you sleep?							
Did you have any dreams/nightmares or other night-time events?							
Did you nap in the day?							

How many hours do you sleep at night on average?_____

Are you satisfied with the amount and quality of sleep you get? _____

Why? _____

Do you wake refreshed, feeling as though you have had enough quality sleep? _____

Refer to the chapter 'Sleep' on page 116.

DIET

For this section, keep an accurate food diary and record everything (yes, everything) you eat and drink over a seven-day period.

A food diary can be as simple as a plain notepad, whether paper or electronic, or you can set up a spreadsheet or download an app. The main thing is that you write down exactly what you eat and drink *at the time*, then and there.

This should be recorded during a period of time when you are in a normal schedule of work and socialising. If your schedule is interrupted – for example, you go on a business trip – then you need to keep a separate record of those meals and transfer them to your diary to get an accurate assessment of potential problem areas.

FOOD DIARY

	MON	TUES	WED	THUR	FRI	SAT	SUN
Breakfast							
Other food/drink consumed in the morning							
Lunch							
Other food/drink consumed in the afternoon							
Dinner							
Other food/drink consumed in the evening							

Refer to the chapter 'Nutrition' on page 132.

MEDICATIONS

On this list note down ANY:

- *prescribed medications,*
- *over the counter preparations,*
- *supplements and*
- *herbal medicines and combinations.*

You will need to go through your medicine cabinet, first-aid kit, bedside tables, kitchen and pantry, handbags and briefcase to see what is in your house, car and office. While you are doing that, discard any medications that are out of date or that you do not expect to take.

Include brand names and generic names, doses and how often you take them. Note whether the strength is in mg, ug or IU.

Include all medications, whether regular or occasional, such as headache tablets that you take only occasionally.

Do you ever take more than the prescribed or recommended amounts? YES/NO

PRESCRIBED MEDICATIONS

NAME	STRENGTH	HOW OFTEN	REASON

OVER THE COUNTER PREPARATIONS

NAME	STRENGTH	HOW OFTEN	REASON

HERBAL MEDICINES AND COMBINATIONS

NAME	STRENGTH	HOW OFTEN	REASON

Refer to the section on pharmaceutical drugs, vitamins and herbal medicines on page 228.

ILLICIT DRUGS

Do you use illicit drugs? YES/NO

Which one(s)? _____

Has your use of illicit drugs caused problems for you personally, at home or at work, or caused problems for others? _____

Have you had trouble with the law? _____

Refer to the chapter 'Illicit drugs' on page 104.

TOXINS

This list may look exhaustive but it is necessary. There will be a discussion later in the book explaining toxins and detox in depth. Some of these questions are also asked in other sections but it is important for you to note the impact of your answers in relation to this particular area.

Do you smoke cigarettes or cannabis? YES/NO

Are you taking any prescribed pharmaceutical drugs? YES/NO

Are you taking any over the counter pharmaceutical preparations? YES/NO

Are you using any recreational drugs? YES/NO

Do you drink alcohol? If so, how often do you drink and how much? YES/NO_____

Have you been exposed to any toxic chemicals in the workplace? This might include a wide variety of occupations, including hairdresser, nail technician, gardener, cleaner, construction worker, painter, farmer, etc. _____

Do you use any pesticides in the house or at work? This would include domestic fly sprays and surface insect sprays, garden pesticides and agricultural chemicals. _____

Do you eat meat or chicken that is not organically farmed? _____

What foods do you eat that are processed and contain preservatives and other additives? Check labels for chemical content of packaged or processed foods. _____

Do you eat fast foods? _____

Which household cleaning products do you use? Are there less toxic choices? _____

Do you have any plastic food or drink containers containing Bisphenol A?

_____

Which cosmetic products do you use, including nail polish, shampoo, perfumes, moisturisers (especially those containing parabens)?

_____

Have you had any dental work involving mercury amalgam? _____

Do you live in an area with high pollution levels? _____

Does your home have an attached garage? YES/NO _____

If yes, do you run the car, lawn mower or other machinery in the garage? Are there adequate seals between the garage and the interior of the house? Is there adequate ventilation? Are potentially toxic items stored in the garage? Are they kept in containers with tightly sealed lids?

_____

Is your bowel function regular or are you constipated? (Optimal gut function is necessary for effective detoxing.) _____

Do you have unchecked sources of stress in your life? _____

Refer to the chapter 'Detox' on page 51.

EXERCISE

Like your food and alcohol diary, keep a diary of the amount of exercise you do. This might include walking the dog, playing a game of tennis or

golf, gardening, taking a dance class or working out at the gym. How much time do you spend outdoors each week?
Refer to the chapter 'Exercise' on page 171.

EXERCISE DIARY

DAY	TYPE	TIME	INTENSITY
MONDAY			
TUESDAY			
WEDNESDAY			
THURSDAY			
FRIDAY			
SATURDAY			
SUNDAY			

SMOKING

Do you smoke? YES/NO
If YES:
How many per day and per week? _____
Do you consider yourself a 'social' or 'occasional' smoker? _____
Are you a regular (most days) smoker? _____
Have you attempted to quit? YES/NO
How many times have you tried to quit and using what methods? _____

_____
If you are an ex-smoker, when did you quit? _____
Refer to the chapter 'Smoking' on page 79.

ALCOHOL

Over an average week, and referring to your food diary, record the number of standard drinks you consume. Remember that a bottle of wine contains 8 standard drinks. A single nip of spirits is equivalent to one standard drink.

ALCOHOL DIARY

DAY	No. of STANDARD alcoholic drinks over a 24-hour period
MON	
TUES	
WED	
THUR	
FRI	
SAT	
SUN	

Average 1–5 drinks per week (low risk) _____

Average 5–10 drinks per week _____

Average more than 10 drinks per week _____

More than 4 drinks in any 24-hour period _____

Has alcohol ever caused any problems in your work, social or
family life? _____

Do you consider alcohol a problem for you now?_____

Refer to the chapter 'Alcohol' on page 67.

EMOTIONAL WELLBEING

There are a number of self-assessment questionnaires for emotional well-being. One of the best known assessment tools is the Kessler Psychological Distress Scale, or K10. Select the response that reflects your feelings over the past two weeks. Then add up your score.

		None of the time (1 point)	A little of the time (2 point)	Some of the time (3 point)	Most of the time (4 point)	All of the time (5 point)
1.	In the past 4 weeks, about how often did you feel tired out for no good reason?					
2.	In the past 4 weeks, about how often did you feel nervous?					

		None of the time (1 point)	A little of the time (2 point)	Some of the time (3 point)	Most of the time (4 point)	All of the time (5 point)
3.	In the past 4 weeks, about how often did you feel so nervous that nothing could calm you down?					
4.	In the past 4 weeks, about how often did you feel hopeless?					
5.	In the past 4 weeks, about how often did you feel restless or fidgety?					
6.	In the past 4 weeks, about how often did you feel so restless you could not sit still?					
7.	In the past 4 weeks, about how often did you feel depressed?					
8.	In the past 4 weeks, about how often did you feel that everything was an effort?					
9.	In the past 4 weeks, about how often did you feel so sad that nothing could cheer you up?					
10.	In the past 4 weeks, about how often did you feel worthless?					
	Total					

Source: Kessler and Mroczek (1994). School of Survey Research Center of the Institute for Social Research. University of Michigan. As cited by Beyond Blue, 2 October 2012, www.beyondblue.org.au.

Lower scores mean a higher degree of emotional health. Higher scores means you need to pay attention to aspects of your emotional health. Talk to your doctor if your score over 20. You can rate your general level of emotional wellbeing, but it is also important to look more closely at some of the influences that impact on your emotional world.

Have you ever had professional counselling or psychotherapy? YES/NO

If YES, why? _____

_____

Has that issue been resolved or is it ongoing? _____

Do you have a partner or spouse? YES/NO

RATE YOUR PRIMARY RELATIONSHIP

	Absolutely not true (1 point)	Occasionally (2 point)	Some of the time (3 point)	Most of the time (4 point)	Absolutely true (5 point)
My partner really cares about me.					
My partner understands the way I feel about things.					
My partner appreciates me.					
I can rely on my partner for help with any serious problem.					
I can openly talk to my partner about my worries.					
I feel completely relaxed and at ease around my partner.					

These scores are just an indicator but they can still be quite revealing.

0-6   You should seriously consider whether to continue this relationship as it is affecting your wellness.

7-18   Your relationship could probably do with some professional help.

19-25 No crisis, but you would benefit from some work on your relationship

24-30 Your relationship is contributing positively to your wellness.

❧ WHO IS AT HOME WITH YOU?

Are there any significant sources of conflict or distress?
List and describe them.

_____

_____

_____

Have you or your close family members experienced any recent major life changes or losses?

_____

_____

_____

WORK

How would you describe your work? _____

1. Can't wait to get there every morning and can't imagine doing anything I would enjoy more.
2. Work is challenging and enjoyable but is really just a means to an end.
3. I would rather be doing something else.
4. I dread walking through the door and can't wait for the weekend.

From these general statements, you can get a sense of your satisfaction at work. Take some time to record more of your own thoughts on your work environment.

_____

_____

WHAT ARE YOUR LEISURE ACTIVITIES/HOBBIES?

1. _____
2. _____

3. _____

4. _____

5. _____

RATE YOUR OVERALL LEVEL OF SATISFACTION OUT OF 5

	1	2	3	4	5
School/university/job					
Social life/friends					
Leisure activities/hobbies					
Home life					
Intimacy/sex					
Children					
Parents/extended family					

Looking at the rating on the table above, you should be able to clearly see which areas of your life are satisfactory and unsatisfactory for you. Refer to the chapters 'Connection' on page 193 and 'Stress and mental health' on page 90.

DIGESTION

Describe your bowel function:

Has there been any recent sustained change in your bowel habit?_____

What is the consistency? Are your stools well-formed/watery/hard/
  variable? _____

How often do you open your bowels?_____

Is there any blood? If so, is it bright or dark? _____

Do you suffer abdominal bloating?_____

Do you pass excessive gas? _____

Do you suffer from heartburn, indigestion or dyspepsia?_____

OTHER SPECIFIC SYMPTOMS AND SIGNS

There are literally hundreds of different symptoms to describe unpleasant physical sensations. Do you experience any of the symptoms below?

☐ pain   ☐ coughing

☐ wheezing   ☐ trouble breathing

- ☐ swelling
- ☐ palpitations
- ☐ nausea
- ☐ urinary incontinence
- ☐ swollen ankles
- ☐ lump
- ☐ loss of appetite
- ☐ frequent urination
- ☐ abnormal bleeding
- ☐ dizziness

_____

_____

_____

_____

NON-SPECIFIC SYMPTOMS

Do you experience symptoms that have not been investigated or diagnosed?
- ☐ fatigue
- ☐ headaches
- ☐ loss of appetite
- ☐ loss of libido
- ☐ excess gas
- ☐ irregular bowel motions
- ☐ abdominal cramps
- ☐ frequent infections
- ☐ rashes

Record the symptoms and other features such as their severity, duration, timing, what makes it better, what makes it worse.

_____

_____

_____

Step 2

REBOOT

Choosing the Right Health Professionals

Detox

Reboot Your Lifestyle
Your Reboot Approach, Alcohol, Smoking, Stress and Mental Health,
Illicit Drugs, Sleep, Nutrition, Food Intolerance and Food Allergy,
Exercise, Immunity, Connection

Integrative Medicine and Complementary Treatments
Acupuncture and Physical Therapies, Taking the Right Pharmaceutical Drugs,
Herbal Medicine, Vitamins and Nutritional Supplements

Choosing the right health professionals

IF YOU ARE THE CAPTAIN, WHO ARE YOUR NAVIGATORS?

To achieve ultimate wellness, you will need the right navigators. As part of your Health Audit, you should audit not only yourself but also those professionals you are trusting to help you solve specific health problems or maintain your general wellbeing. You need to gather a team of healthcare professionals with the right skills and attitudes to help you achieve your health goals.

One of the reasons why I became so interested in the field of integrative medicine is that it provides a way to harness the many methods of finding solutions to health problems. The health sector is broad and varied in its philosophies and skills. By choosing the right type of practitioner with the right skills at the right time, you will minimise confusion and fast-track your way to where you want to go with your wellbeing.

In this chapter I will discuss the importance of your general practitioner (GP) and advise you on other health professionals you may consult to help you achieve ultimate wellbeing.

WHY YOU NEED A GP YOU CAN TRUST

I will declare my interest up front: I am a doctor, a specialist in general practice and I strongly believe that a regular GP is a non-negotiable prerequisite to your comprehensive health care.

It is not enough to see a non-medical practitioner only for 'wellness visits' without having regular medical check-ups, even if you think you have no specific medical problems. Only doctors are fully trained in detection and diagnosis of the warning signs of disease. Our training is carefully focused on getting the diagnosis right. You can't get that by just talking, or having your pulse taken or from someone looking into your eyes.

Your doctor is going to be able to take a comprehensive medical history, do *all* of the physical examinations that might be required (especially the more invasive or intimate ones), refer for appropriate investigations, make a medical diagnosis and formulate a comprehensive treatment plan. This is the reason why I am so insistent that people find a GP or family physician they trust and see them regularly, preferably annually.

Ideally, your doctor will have a good working knowledge of the range of allied and complementary therapies that interest you or would benefit you, and be able to guide you in an informed way to the therapies that have the best chance of working for you with the lowest risk of adverse effects.

There are some health commentators who criticise this approach as 'doctor-centric'. I make no apology for this. In my experience, it is the safest model to ensure that most basic of health principles: finding out whether anything is wrong that needs to be addressed medically, and then formulating the best and safest approach to getting you well.

The right doctor for you:

* makes you feel comfortable to discuss any problem
* listens to you without making you feel rushed
* does not make you feel judged
* takes a thorough medical history and examines you
* shares or respects your health philosophy
* demonstrates a depth of knowledge and skill about issues of importance to you
* leaves you feeling confident
* has consulting rooms which feel comfortable and efficiently managed
* refers you appropriately to allied health practitioners or medical specialists

SO HOW DO YOU GO ABOUT CHOOSING THE DOCTOR WHO IS RIGHT FOR YOU?

If you have a GP you like and trust, and who shares your philosophy of health care, then problem solved. If you don't, then what do you look for in a doctor? You need someone who makes you feel comfortable, and who you feel listens. You clearly need to be satisfied that the doctor has a depth of knowledge and skill about issues of importance to you.

Once you have spent a little time on your Health Audit, you will develop a clearer idea of the priority areas for you. Your GP will likely ask you a lot of questions along the lines of the Health Audit, but because you have had the opportunity to assess your own priorities, you know in what areas you need some specific testing or are seeking advice. Your GP is also perfectly placed to monitor your progress with you and, where necessary, navigate you towards other appropriate health professionals or medical specialists.

If you have specific health issues then you may also need one or more medical specialists as consultants in their relevant fields of expertise. The important thing is that you have the right team, and that they are all talking to each other.

♣ COMMUNICATION

The protocols for doctors to communicate with each other are well established. The GP writes a letter to the specialist covering all your relevant information, including your medications and medical history. The specialist sees you and writes back to the GP with the results of any investigations or treatments and their opinion. Hospitals ideally, but not always, send a discharge summary to the GP so that they know if you have been admitted to hospital, and they also provide them with any changes to your medical treatment and requests for follow-up.

Other health practitioners tend to be less consistent with their communication. The GP might or might not hear about your visit to the physiotherapist or podiatrist.

Communication can be a particular problem where there are professional, language or cultural differences. For example, a Traditional Chinese Medicine (TCM) practitioner may find it difficult to communicate with a Western trained doctor, as they may not understand each other's professional terminology. This can be overcome, but it can be difficult. For a Western trained doctor, having a patient come in and say, 'My acupuncturist said I have low qi in my kidney meridian', might be confusing if the terminology is not familiar to them.

What is impossible is when one of the health professionals you see is just not interested in what your other health professionals have to say, or has no respect for their expertise. I know this puts some people off even mentioning other treatments they are having.

Ideally your various health professionals will work well together. If your team isn't able to or willing to communicate effectively, then you need to look around and put together a team that will.

CONSOLIDATING YOUR MEDICAL RECORDS

I encourage every one of my patients to consolidate their medical records. Because I do a lot of case reviews, I often see patients who have already seen multiple doctors, specialists and other practitioners and had masses of investigations but have not found a satisfactory answer to their health problems. Although I ask new patients to bring along all their results and reports, we often have to spend considerable time tracking down original pathology or CT scan results and specialist reports.

All it takes is a ring folder that can hold transparent plastic sleeves, a little assertiveness and a tiny bit of organisational skill. To start with, ask your GP to provide you with a health summary, which is usually just one or two sheets of paper with a summary of relevant details, such as past medical history, current medications and supplements, allergies and immunisations. This is very simple if your GP has computerised records.

Ask to be copied in to any blood tests, and file copies of any investigation reports. Then ask your specialists if you can be provided with copies of their reports, including investigations, procedures and opinions. Often I find patients do not know the results of their original tests and are unclear about exactly what they were treated for and why.

The same goes for any allied health practitioners and complementary medicine practitioners. It is not possible for me to work out a comprehensive summary with a patient if I do not know what supplements or herbal treatments or other treatment modalities they have tried, whether successfully or unsuccessfully, or are currently using. If I can see a precise list of ingredients, then I can work out what doses and combinations they are taking and whether there are any potential interactions or risks of adverse events.

HOW YOUR GP RELATES TO OTHER HEALTH PROFESSIONALS

You will encounter GPs and specialists at various levels of enlightenment when it comes to complementary treatments, varying according to their training or education in aspects of complementary therapies and their general attitude to them. If you feel you want to explore complementary medicine treatments alongside your medical treatment then you will test a GP for openness and for how competently they discuss your options.

They may be:

- *uninformed and openly hostile*
- *interested but uninformed*
- *informed and encouraging of safe and effective treatments while warning appropriately of unsafe or ineffective treatments.*

Fortunately, the second group is growing – the doctors who are interested but uninformed – as is the third. Most GPs are definitely interested in knowing more about complementary medicines.

RATES OF PRACTICE AND REFERRAL FOR COMPLEMENTARY THERAPIES BY AUSTRALIAN GPs.

	Ever referred (%)	Have practised (%)
acupuncture	89.6	19.0
meditation	79.6	15.3
hypnosis	81.6	8.7
chiropractic	68.5	5.0
herbal medicine	29.1	4.8
naturopathy	29.7	3.2
vitamin therapy	16.9	25.1
homeopathy	19.2	2.5
osteopathy	29.6	2.8
aromatherapy	17.5	1.1
spiritual healing	19.5	2.1
reflexology	10.1	0.5

Source: MV Pirotta, MM Cohen, V Kotsirilos et al., 'Complementary therapies: have they become accepted in general practice?', Medical Journal of Australia, 2007; 172(3): pp. 105–109

An interesting survey of Australian GPs in 2005 found that over 75 per cent of GPs said they formally refer their patients for complementary therapies, so it is definitely becoming mainstream practice.

Some doctors who practise integrative medicine have done postgraduate study to develop skills in one or other forms of complementary medicine, such as nutritional medicine, acupuncture or hypnotherapy. Others practise primarily by providing the conventional medical therapies themselves, and referring to or interacting with a variety of providers of complementary therapies.

The therapies with particularly high referral rates by GPs are acupuncture, meditation, hypnosis and chiropractic. Herbal medicine, naturopathy and osteopathy also have referral rates of close to 30 per cent. In terms of doctors practising complementary therapies, vitamin therapy is most frequently used, followed by acupuncture, meditation and hypnosis.

There is what I call a hierarchy of acceptance of complementary therapies by doctors. This tends to be closely related to the doctor's knowledge of the treatment and its perceived risks and benefits. Treatments that doctors perceive have the lowest risk of adverse effects tend to be lowest on the scale of controversy. This might include massage, tai chi, sensible dietary modification, or aromatherapy. You will see higher levels of controversy with interventions such as herbal medicine, intravenous vitamin therapy and acupuncture.

The other factor in medical acceptance of a therapy is the level of plausibility of the particular treatment, and whether there has been research to show that it works. For example, while homeopathy has a negligible risk of adverse effects, it has become very controversial in the United Kingdom and Australia because it is perceived as 'implausible' and because there is very sparse evidence that it works.

Conversely, we also run into difficulty when there is reasonable or even substantial scientific evidence for a therapy but it has not percolated through into the literature that doctors routinely access, and the bodies that advise doctors do not look at these sources of information to include in treatment protocols and guidelines.

Doctors who define themselves as 'integrative medicine practitioners' generally have a wider frame of reference for seeking information. Unfortunately, despite the increasing prevalence of use of complementary medicine and the growing interest in integrative medicine, medical education in universities and specialist colleges in Australia has been slow to incorporate these topics into the curriculum.

OTHER HEALTH PROFESSIONALS

Doctors do not have all the answers, nor can we be all things to all people; hence the need to choose the right types of allied health professionals for your health advice and treatment. Hopefully your GP can assist you to navigate the system by investigating and diagnosing your problem to work out which other health professionals are appropriate for you.

Other health professionals include:

- dentist
- nurse/nurse practitioner
- physiotherapist
- chiropractor
- osteopath
- massage therapist
- podiatrist (feet)
- audiologist (ears)
- optometrist (eyes)
- psychologist (mind)
- counsellor
- social worker
- dietitian (nutrition)
- exercise physiologist
- personal trainer
- occupational therapist
- speech pathologist
- naturopath
- herbalist
- TCM practitioner
- acupuncturist
- pharmacist
- homeopath

There are great advantages to getting timely and credible advice. But there are great potential risks and expense involved in pursuing treatments that are inappropriate, ineffective or, at worst, dangerous.

First and foremost, the practitioner needs to be well trained. When you see a doctor, you know that they have attained a specific level of education and that they have compulsory continuing professional development. With other types of practitioners, it helps when there is a system of professional registration and regulation. That means that the profession has agreed on minimum standards for training, education and continuing professional development, and that an independent regulatory body is responsible for upholding those professional standards.

This administration of standards applies to most healthcare professions, including medicine, nursing, physiotherapy, podiatry, audiology, dietetics, psychology and so on. Some practitioners will have special postgraduate training in a particularly specialised area of their profession. For example, some physiotherapists have further training in the treatment of spinal problems or rehabilitation.

In the field of natural therapies there is a wide variation in training and knowledge. TCM in Australia took many years to gain recognition, but registration went national in 2012. However some professions or philosophies of health care do not fall under any scheme of professional registration and regulation, which makes it difficult to choose a practitioner. This also makes it difficult for the registered professions to interact with those who are not registered, for safety reasons as well as for medico-legal reasons.

This situation will change with time because professional groups such as naturopaths and herbalists have recognised this as a problem for consumers and for the standing of responsible practitioners, and they are actively seeking a system of registration.

WHO IS THE RIGHT PRACTITIONER FOR YOU TO SEE?

Some doctors have undertaken further study to gain skills in one or more aspects of complementary medicine, such as acupuncture or nutritional medicine. Your doctor may be able to point you in the right direction and refer you directly to another practitioner because they will have assessed the training and skills of the other practitioner and be aware of their areas of special interest.

Doctors also listen to feedback from patients who tell us of their experiences with practitioners, both positive and negative. If you would like to see a particular practitioner, you may be able to discuss their suitability with your GP.

If you are doing your own research, you will need to ask the practitioner directly or check their website for their qualifications. If necessary, track down the institution that granted the qualification and find out what the course entails in terms of time and content, and whether it is a certificate, diploma or degree course.

But be aware that even this is not a guarantee of the right skills to suit your needs. For example, a person might have a science degree or a nursing degree from a university (or no degree at all) and call themselves a naturopath without having trained as one.

Sometimes you will be relying on the recommendation of friends or relatives or some other source to see a practitioner.

Whichever non-medical practitioner you see, it should immediately ring alarm bells if they discourage you in any way from continuing care with your GP or medical specialists.

❧ CHOOSING A NATUROPATH OR HERBALIST

A naturopath is a health practitioner who uses nutritional and lifestyle advice, herbs and supplements and sometimes other techniques such as massage with the aim of supporting or boosting the body's natural healing ability. If you want to visit a naturopath, I strongly advise you to first visit your GP or medical specialist to make sure you have the correct diagnosis, and to ensure you are not missing something. Naturopathy is not strong on medical diagnosis, so it works best in situations where you have already had a diagnosis and you want to augment your medical treatment with lifestyle changes and natural therapies. Alternatively, if you have been medically checked and a specific diagnosis has been ruled out, you might want help to regain your wellbeing with a focus on lifestyle modification, nutrition and natural therapies.

So-called complementary medicine (CM) has been under attack from the forces of medical conservatism in recent times. Naturopaths and herbalists form one of the largest and most often consulted groups of CM practitioners, but with all that controversy, should you be thinking about seeing a naturopath at all? If so, how do you choose the right practitioner for you?

Despite the popularity of naturopathy with the public there is no system of registration for practitioners in Australia, so there is no minimum level of education or professional standards. This creates a problem if you want to see a naturopath, because while some naturopaths are highly qualified, someone can set up practice with very little or no training at all. There is also no national code of conduct, nowhere you can complain if there is a problem and no disciplinary process for inappropriate or dangerous activity in the way that, say, the medical profession is monitored.

So how do you choose? If your doctor practices integrative medicine, then it is likely they will have assessed the qualifications of some naturopaths in your area and will be able to point you in the right direction. Otherwise you will need to ask questions yourself about the practitioner's qualifications and check out the educational standard of the institution that provided the course.

Find out what the naturopath charges. The cost of consultations is very variable. Medicare does not provide any subsidy for visits to naturopaths, but some private health fund policies will subsidise visits to naturopaths who are members of their professional association.

The cost can escalate when supplements or herbs are prescribed and dispensed. These can be expensive, particularly if a number of supplements are recommended. Do not feel obliged to buy all the supplements that are recommended by the naturopath. Ask exactly what is being prescribed and why, and where you can find evidence for their efficacy in your condition.

Can naturopaths hinder you?

The main precaution with seeing a naturopath or other CM practitioner is to make sure you are not discouraged from following your medical advice. You should hear alarm bells if you are promised some kind of unrealistic or 'miraculous' cure.

If you see a naturopath or other CM practitioner, ask for scientific evidence of any therapies they recommend, and check whether there are any interactions with medications you are taking.

Choosing a naturopath

- Look for a degree from a reputable university or college.
- Ensure the naturopath is a member of a professional association such as the National Herbalists Association of Australia.
- Ask friends, family and other health practitioners for personal recommendations.
- Find out if the naturopath has expertise with your particular health issue.
- Ask whether the naturopath will communicate with your doctor, especially if you have a chronic or serious medical condition.
- Choose someone who is prepared to explain the reason for any supplements or herbs they suggest you take.
- Beware of extravagant promises.
- Find out if the practitioner is covered by your private health fund.

It is essential that you tell your GP when you are taking herbs or supplements prescribed by a naturopath or herbalist, and make sure you tell your naturopath or herbalist the full list of medications you are taking. Anyone prescribing or recommending treatments for you has to know all the other medications or supplements you are taking because you need to avoid the risk of an adverse interaction.

It would be fair to say that the medical profession has mixed feelings about naturopaths. From my point of view as an integrative medicine doctor, a naturopath who is highly trained in herbal and nutritional therapies, understands herb–drug interactions and communicates with your medical team is a valuable addition to your healthcare team.

Someone who calls themselves a naturopath but does not have the appropriate education can give you inaccurate or dangerous advice, waste your time and money, interfere with appropriate medical treatments and have a negative effect on your health.

Dietitian, naturopath or nutritionist?

How do you tell the difference between a dietician, a nutritionist and a naturopath? A naturopath or a nutritionist may give you advice about diet and nutrition, but the term 'dietitian' refers to a university-trained and registered Accredited Practising Dietitian (APD) focusing on the role of nutrition in health. This would be the most appropriate professional to see if you have a significant health problem where nutrition is a factor in the cause or the treatment. Examples might be eating disorders, obesity, diabetes, inflammatory bowel disease, cancer and so on. Generally speaking, dietitians do not focus much on nutritional supplementation, while a naturopath may recommend nutritional supplements and herbal medicines.

Then there are the health professionals called 'nutritionists'. There is no minimum qualification to use this term. A nutritionist has generally completed a diploma course, not a university course, and the quality of training varies wildly. In fact, you do not need to have had any formal training at all to call yourself a nutritionist.

If you need specialised nutrition advice, your best bet is a university-qualified and registered dietitian. In Australia, Medicare rebates may be available with a referral from a doctor. For advice on nutrition and nutritional supplements, herbal medicines and herb–drug interactions, a well-trained naturopath would be the right person to see.

❦ ACUPUNCTURIST

Not all acupuncturists are doctors and not all doctors practise acupuncture. Another point of difference is that a TCM practitioner will also prescribe Chinese herbal medicines, whereas a Western trained doctor who is trained in acupuncture usually does not.

From 2012, TCM practitioners have been registered nationally as a profession in Australia. That does not guarantee a practitioner will have a comprehensive university education, as some practitioners have been 'grandfathered' onto the register because they have been working as TCM practitioners for many years. To make sure that the practitioner you are seeing has a minimum level of qualification, check whether they have graduated from a reputable university and if they are registered with their appropriate professional body to practise acupuncture.

These days it should go without saying, but also ensure that the practitioner uses new disposable needles that are discarded after each treatment.

❦ PHYSIOTHERAPIST, OSTEOPATH OR CHIROPRACTOR?

A common quandary I face is where to refer people who need musculo-skeletal therapy, particularly for neck and back pain. Sometimes it is an easy call to make. In other cases you may need to try one type of treatment to see if it is likely to be effective or not, as there is a lot of crossover between the treatment types.

A physiotherapist will do a biomechanical and ergonomic – posture and movement – assessment. Treatment may include manual hands-on therapy, such as massage or gentle tissue manipulation, exercise therapy, ergonomic advice and taping. They may use machines such as ultrasound or transcutaneous electrical nerve stimulation (TENS).

You will be given advice regarding how to manage any injury and possibly some exercises to do at home or at work.

A physiotherapist can help to:

- *decrease pain from injury*
- *restore normal range of joint movement*
- *improve muscle and joint function*
- *facilitate return to sport after injury*
- *assist with post-operative rehabilitation.*

Both physiotherapists and osteopaths work on soft tissue and the function of the muscles and skeleton. They offer treatment for conditions such as headache, back pain, muscle and joint strain and stiffness, and injuries.

Chiropractic, in brief, is based on the theory that health and wellbeing is related to proper spinal column position and condition. Treatment consists of a range of manipulative techniques, mostly on the spine.

You can see any of these practitioners without a medical referral, but consider seeing your doctor first, or if treatment is not helping your progress. In the case of musculoskeletal problems or sports injuries, an opinion from a sports physician (a doctor specialising in musculoskeletal medicine) can help to direct you. Diagnosis and advice will be an important part of your decision.

Your choice of practitioner will depend on the nature of your problem at a particular time and the philosophy of care you feel sits most comfortably with you.

❧ EXERCISE PHYSIOLOGIST OR PERSONAL TRAINER?

An exercise physiologist is an allied health professional who specialises in using exercise as part of the treatment for patients with a medical condition. They can prescribe a course of exercises for either fitness or rehabilitation. Exercise physiologists complete a university degree and have wide knowledge about the workings of the human body and the physical and mental effects of exercise on it. They differ from a personal trainer (PT) at the gym, who would be more accurately described as a fitness professional.

The education of personal trainers varies considerably and their focus is on fitness, motivation and the technical accuracy of exercises. You can call yourself a personal trainer with no qualifications. Some have done brief courses of a few weeks while others are more experienced, and the better quality gyms ensure their PTs are suitably qualified. I strongly advise you to check the qualifications of a PT before undertaking a training program.

If you have a significant medical problem such as diabetes, heart disease, arthritis, back pain, asthma or osteoporosis, or you are recovering from an injury or illness, then it would be wise to have your exercise program carefully worked out and supervised by an exercise physiologist.

Some stress can be solved by assessing your life, viewing things from a different angle and deciding to make positive changes. You can also find it constructive talking to your partner, a friend, a mentor or work colleagues. But there are times when the best approach is to call for specialised professional help.

After you complete your Health Audit and read the information in the 'Stress and mental health' chapter on page 90, you may wish to seek further support from a mental health professional. When I talk to patients about being referred to a specialist in this area, they are often unsure about the difference between a psychiatrist and a psychologist, and it can be confusing.

Psychologists and psychiatrists both work in the area of mental health, so they help with emotional and psychological problems, and also help people without a diagnosed mental health condition to improve their emotional health or manage relationship difficulties that might be impacting on their emotions. Even within these disciplines there is a wide variation in the type of training and expertise in specialised areas.

To become a psychiatrist you first have to complete a medical degree. This is then followed by several years of specialist training and supervised clinical experience. A psychiatrist will engage in some type of 'talk therapy' and, being a doctor, a psychiatrist can prescribe medication such as antidepressants and antipsychotic drugs where they consider them necessary.

A psychologist has specialised clinical training in non-pharmaceutical interventions such as cognitive behaviour therapy and other techniques for psychological problems and maintaining mental health. The pathway to becoming a registered psychologist differs somewhat from country to country. In Australia, a psychologist must complete a four-year undergraduate degree followed by two years of supervised clinical experience or completion of a clinical masters degree or doctorate in clinical psychology.

There are many types of counsellors and they may have training as a psychologist or come from a nursing or social work background. Counsellors may have special expertise in a particular area, such as relationships, career advice, fertility, parenting, drug and alcohol addiction, sexual abuse, cancer, stress management or grief. If you are going to see a counsellor, you will need to check out their qualifications and experience, and their areas of special interest and training to see if they are suitable to help you with your problem.

HOW ABOUT ANOTHER OPINION?

The question of second opinions comes up all the time in medical practice. The most common type you may be familiar with is the referral to a specialist in a particular area of expertise, such as a dermatologist for a skin problem or a cardiologist for a heart problem. Usually this is because your GP knows that they need the opinion of an expert who is focused on a particular disease or body part. Most GPs will have a very good sense of when it is appropriate to ask for a specialist opinion.

A lot of my patients talk to me about second opinions from additional specialists. Sometimes I see a patient for the first time because they have not been happy with the way their health has been managed so far, in which case I am the one being asked for a second opinion. In some cases it turns out to be a third, fourth or fifth opinion if there has been a long search for answers.

There are advantages and disadvantages to seeking extra opinions. Medical diagnosis and health care is not always an exact science, and sometimes medical conditions can be very complicated. So if you are in a situation where you are not making progress, it makes sense to get a fresh perspective.

People are often reluctant to hurt 'their' doctor's feelings, and I understand this. The way the health system in Australia works makes it relatively easy to seek second opinions. If you feel you want a different GP's perspective then you just need to make an appointment, take along as many results of your blood tests, scans and specialist reports as you can get hold of and go to see another GP. The downside here is that some tests may be repeated unnecessarily and there is a loss of continuity of care. This is another advantage of maintaining a file with as many of your results and reports as possible.

In a group general practice, with all of the patients' records in the one location, we are accustomed to the possibility of patients seeing various practitioners in the group from time to time and that does often bring a new perspective. But I have come across doctors who have felt threatened or annoyed by patients seeking other opinions. Really, that is just too bad. Your health is the most important priority.

If you do want a second opinion from a specialist or other health practitioner, then you can discuss that with your GP. They will need to be satisfied both professionally and ethically that the second opinion is in your best interest.

Where you might run into trouble is if you get so many conflicting opinions that treatment becomes confusing and then you can become paralysed by indecision, not knowing who to trust or what to do. A common scenario is the person who is diagnosed with cancer and chemotherapy is recommended by their cancer specialist (oncologist). They then see several other oncologists who recommend different types of treatment protocol, or advise against chemotherapy, and then the patient and their well-meaning friends and family consult Dr Google and become completely bamboozled by the different advice they gather. Add to that the majority of patients who use some form of complementary therapies during their cancer treatment and do not tell their oncologist or GP what else they are doing, and the result is a recipe for confusion and potential danger.

❧ THE INTERNET

Case study

Susan came to see me with a 'rabbit caught in the headlights' expression on her face. She had requested an urgent appointment.

Before she even sat down, she said, 'I have MS.'

'MS?' I repeated. 'As in multiple sclerosis?'

'Yes. I figured it out from the internet. I googled my symptoms and that's what came up.'

Start with the basics, I thought. Breathe. 'So, what are your symptoms?'

'Well, I have this weird tingling in my left arm that comes and goes, and sometimes my arm feels weak.'

To cut a long story short, a physical examination and a couple of physiotherapy treatments later, the tingling from a nerve entrapment in her neck disappeared. Not MS at all.

I mentioned Dr Google. This is because the internet is an omnipresence in medical consultations these days, and pretty much every patient I know has jumped onto the web to do a search about their symptoms or their condition or their medication. Seeking reliable information is a great idea. For a GP, however, it is a double-edged sword.

As a patient or 'health consumer', arming yourself with information is a crucial part of good decision making. But if the information is questionable, or voluminous, or confusing, or not directly related to your specific current situation, it can waste a lot of your time and also cause unnecessary panic.

Not all websites are reliable or accurate and so you really need to be careful where you find information, and that it comes from a credible source. Some websites are brilliant but others are plain irresponsible and wrong.

On the positive side, I learn a lot from patients who are motivated to spend the time finding new information that may not have hit our medical news yet. Where that helps your healthcare decisions, it is always very welcome.

This also gets back to making sure you have the right team of health professionals in place. You can ask them about reliable and credible websites. Then using the internet to gain more information about your condition is a value-add.

Detox

Once you have completed your Health Audit and identified the areas in your life that need the most change, you are ready for the phase we will call your 'detox'.

How often do you hear someone say, 'I'm going to do a detox'? It seems to be the plan *du jour* for people who recognise they are not feeling as well or as energetic as they would like, and decide they need to do something to radically alter their lifestyle, even if it is just a temporary 'flash in the pan' effort. In your pursuit of ultimate wellbeing, it really is worthwhile considering a sensible detox process.

And I stress the word *sensible*.

I want to show you how, with minimal effort and expense, you can work out your own sensible and healthy detox program, and not just for a few weeks but as a transition to a conscious, mindful lifestyle choice that sets up the right conditions for you to feel terrific all the time.

WHAT IS A DETOX?

Let's first be clear about what detox actually means. The aim of a detox is to eliminate as many toxins from your body as possible for as long as possible. 'Detox' is one of those concepts that means different things to different people. For example, for some people it means an extreme process of weeks of water or juice fasting with colonic washes and meditation for 12 hours a day in a health retreat. For others it involves removing anything chemical or processed from their diet and environment for a period of time. Some people want it to just mean not smoking or drinking alcohol or caffeine for a week or two, then going back to their familiar but unhealthy old habits.

There are simple and safe detox processes that you can plan yourself, while more sophisticated or detailed detoxing needs professional advice and supervision by a doctor with training in environmental medicine and complementary therapies. The extent and complexity of a detox will vary depending on your individual health status, needs and preferences. Supervision and professional advice is particularly important if you have a medical condition such as diabetes or kidney disease, or if you have been diagnosed with heavy metal toxicity.

WHAT IS THE 'TOX' IN 'DETOX'?

Detox is short for detoxification, and refers to the removal of harmful or potentially harmful substances that can interact with your body chemistry and affect your health and wellbeing. Unless you live in Antarctica, toxins are almost impossible to avoid completely. Actually, even if you live in Antarctica there will be some toxins in the environment. They are, literally, everywhere.

Your body has natural mechanisms to deal with a certain level of some, but not all, toxins, and the organs responsible for processing and eliminating toxins are the liver, gut, lungs, skin and kidneys. Modern lifestyles in the developed world, and the increase in environmental pollutants through industrialisation, can combine to overwhelm your body's capacity to clear toxins, and they can accumulate in body fluids and tissues, particularly in adipose, or fat, tissue. We are increasingly recognising the link between environmental and dietary toxins and a range of diseases. We are also recognising that toxins can be passed on to the developing foetus through the umbilical cord during pregnancy, and to a baby during breastfeeding.

Some toxins are produced by your body processes. They include:

- *the biochemical end products of stress and negative emotions*
- *some hormones*
- *free radicals from oxidative stress causing premature ageing, and which are associated with diseases such as arthritis and cancer, and immune system disorders.*

The bulk of toxins in the body are related to environmental or dietary exposure. Some of these are easily eliminated, while others are beyond your immediate control. They include:

- *artificial food additives such as some food colourings, flavouring agents and preservatives*
- *pharmaceuticals*
- *lifestyle-related toxins, such as cigarette smoke, alcohol, caffeine and recreational drugs*
- *toxins produced by bacteria*
- *heavy metals, such as lead, mercury, cadmium and aluminium*
- *vehicle exhaust fumes*
- *pesticides used in agriculture and in the home and garden*

- *plasticisers used in packaging, such as phthalates, Bisphenol A*
- *industrial chemicals*
- *household cleaning chemicals.*

HEALTH PROBLEMS RELATED TO TOXIN EXPOSURE OR OVERLOAD

Unless you have been diagnosed with a significant definable disease, the vague and often trivial nature of some of the symptoms of toxin overload can easily be dismissed as inevitable signs of getting older or being overworked or stressed. The consequences of toxin overload on your wellbeing might include a plethora of non-specific symptoms.

Vague or non-specific symptoms of toxin overload

- fatigue
- trouble sleeping
- irritability
- difficulty concentrating
- aches and pains
- bloating
- weight gain
- bad breath
- sore throat
- excess mucus in the nose
- poor complexion.

Research is emerging that increasingly links toxins to a range of not only minor symptoms, but also more serious health issues. This is not a complete list, nor is toxin exposure/overload the one and only explanation or solution for these health issues, but it may form part of the puzzle. The links between diseases and toxins include:

- ***neurology*** – *headaches and migraines, multiple sclerosis, Parkinson's disease, ADHD, Alzheimer's disease*
- ***immunity*** – *some toxins are known to reduce immune function, increasing the risk of infections and cancers. Some environmental agents are known to cause autoimmune-type reactions, such as lupus or lupus-like conditions*
- ***allergy*** – *some toxins are associated with common allergies*
- ***inflammation*** – *some toxins are known to increase the risk of inflammatory conditions such as arthritis, fibromyalgia and musculoskeletal aches and pains*

- *overweight and obesity* – *some toxins alter your body's fat metabolism and energy production mechanisms leading to problems with being overweight*

- *hormonal* – *toxins have been implicated in the risk of premature puberty in girls, infertility or sub-fertility in males and females, premenstrual syndrome, and some hormone-associated cancers such as breast cancer*

- *diabetes* – *there is a possible association between environmental toxins, and the development of type 1 and type 2 diabetes*

- *cancers* – *the* Journal of the American Medical Association *published an opinion that even once smoking is factored out, rates of cancer are higher for those born after 1940 and can be partly attributed to an increased exposure to environmental carcinogens. The* British Medical Journal *agreed, saying that, 'Environmental and lifestyle factors are key determinants of human disease – accounting for perhaps 75 per cent of most cancers'. The mechanism is through the mutation of cells by toxic chemicals.*

- *respiratory* – *indoor and outdoor air pollution is responsible for a higher risk of asthma, chronic bronchitis and respiratory infections.*

It is important not to assume that any of these symptoms or diseases is caused by, or worsened by, toxins in your environment or your diet, or that eliminating them will eliminate the health problem.

A prerequisite to a detox process is to visit your doctor for a comprehensive medical history and examination, appropriate investigation, accurate diagnosis and medical advice, and a discussion about any special precautions. Once you have established whether or not you have a significant medical condition needing specific treatment, you can proceed to the elements of detox as a step to your healthier lifestyle.

If you are taking pharmaceutical medications, your medical appointment is an opportunity to have a medication review. This involves checking the doses and combinations of all of your medicines (prescribed and over the counter) to see what is necessary, what might be causing you problems and what you could safely reduce or eliminate. It is very important for your safety that you do not cease or change medications without guidance from your doctor. I am sometimes asked for an opinion on whether someone can stop their medication or switch it to a non-pharmaceutical option. There will be times when this is possible and safe. Some medications, however, treat or control serious or life-threatening medical problems and carefully targeted and balanced pharmaceutical therapy is the best and safest option.

THE DETOX PROCESS

There are a number of different detox protocols or processes. Generally speaking, detoxing has three stages:
1. identify the toxins
2. eliminate the toxins, and
3. restore balance.

IDENTIFYING TOXINS

The first step in any detox process is to identify the sources of toxins that might be affecting you. When you do this exercise, you may be shocked to see how many chemicals you expose yourself to every day, whether intentionally or unintentionally. Some will be relatively harmless and easily eliminated by your body. But others are not so harmless or easy to eliminate.

Once you have completed your personal toxin audit, you can set about removing as many toxins as possible from every part of your home, your workplace and your lifestyle. The aim is to help to restore your body's own natural capacity to eliminate toxins.

Your personal toxin audit

Go back to the Health Audit Questionnaire (page 15) and review your results in the section marked 'Toxins'. Once you have assessed your potential and actual exposure to toxins in your life, you will know what you need to eliminate.

If, on the basis of your audit you believe that you may have a problem with toxin load, then you can have laboratory tests done to assess the levels of some specific toxins. Laboratory tests can be used to measure the levels of some toxins, assess physiological detoxification pathways and help in coming to the right conclusions. This option needs to be carefully considered, because the tests are costly and many are performed only by a small number of laboratories. You may also find that the tests are not refundable through government or private health insurance.

When doctors decide to order investigations, we need to answer the questions, 'Will this test help me in making an accurate diagnosis?' and 'Will this test help to guide my treatment decisions?' You may also like to ask the question: 'Is this test worth the cost?'

Many accumulated toxins are stored in fat tissue, so blood tests, urine tests and hair analysis will only provide a proxy measurement for the true levels of toxicity. Examples of testing methods include:

- **hair mineral analyses** – *test for heavy metal exposure (for example, mercury, aluminium, arsenic, cadmium) and nutrient deficiency (calcium, magnesium, selenium, zinc, boron). The result reflects your toxin levels over the past 2–3 months. You need to provide samples that have not had any chemical treatment, such as dyeing, because chemical products interfere with the results. Depending on the results, further tests from blood and urine might be arranged.*

- **serum, urine and faecal heavy metal tests** – *measure aluminium, arsenic, cadmium, chromium, lead and mercury. These tests need to be interpreted by an expert.*

- **functional liver tests** – *phase 1 and phase 2 liver detoxification pathways can be assessed by exposing you to metered doses of three toxins – caffeine, paracetamol and aspirin – and measuring the levels of their by-products in blood or urine samples over 24 hours. The results can help pinpoint imbalances in liver detoxification and tailor a treatment plan.*

- **gut dysbiosis tests** – *faeces can be tested for evidence of dysbiosis (imbalance in gut bacteria) or the presence of unhealthy bacteria with a highly specialised analysis.*

THE ELIMINATION PROCESS

Start with the kitchen and check out your fridge and freezer, then the pantry. This is always good for a few surprises. Check nutrition panels for artificial colourings, flavourings and preservatives. While you're at it, throw out anything that has passed its use-by date.

Make sure that you store food in glass or, if you do use plastic, check that it is free of Bisphenol A. Many plastic containers are marked with a triangle with a number in the centre. Higher grade plastics have a number greater than or equal to 5; 7 is ideal. Avoid heating any food in plastic containers.

Then look at your household cleaning products, including dishwashing liquids. Check the chemical ingredients.

The bathroom cabinet is next. Take out all the cosmetics, perfumes, toothpastes and other toiletries. Check the labels for ingredients, especially parabens. If you are serious about a detox, you will also assess the cosmetic products you use and replace as many as possible with products that are chemical free and have natural or organic ingredients.

❧ ELIMINATE TOXINS

Go back to your Health Audit. The areas relating to toxins in your lifestyle are the ones most accessible to change. While you cannot do much about air pollution levels around where you live, there are some actions you can take.

If you have an attached garage, you can make sure the garage is well-ventilated. Ensure there is an effective seal around the door leading into the house. Avoid leaving the ignition on in the car when the door of the garage is closed. Also avoid running any machinery (petrol or diesel driven) in the garage unless the garage door is wide open.

You can also eliminate the pollution you inhale into your lungs from cigarette smoke. If you smoke, now is the time to quit. If you have a smoker in the house who refuses to quit, try to negotiate a smoke-free house. It is rare these days to hear of a household where people smoke indoors, especially if children are living there, but if that is the case in your home, it is something you can change to reduce your toxin load.

If your house has air-conditioning, make sure to have it regularly cleaned by a professional. If you have a combustion heater, consider replacing it to reduce your exposure to carbon monoxide.

❧ VOLATILE ORGANIC COMPOUNDS

Volatile organic compounds (VOCs) are emitted by thousands of different types of products, including cleaning products, disinfectants, floor coverings, office equipment, pesticides, building materials, furnishings, glues, adhesives, permanent markers, paints and lacquers. VOCs are up to ten times higher indoors than outdoors. Exposure to VOCs can cause headaches; eye, nose and throat irritation; loss of coordination; fatigue; nausea; and dizziness. Some VOCs are suspected or known to cause cancer.

You can reduce the VOC load in your home by replacing whatever products you can that contain VOCs with environmentally friendly products. Do not store VOC-containing products in your home. Make sure your home is regularly ventilated with fresh air.

DETOX DIET

A poor diet is high in unhealthy fats, refined carbohydrates and sugar, and food additives such as colourings and preservatives, but low in protein and essential nutrients, such as vitamins and minerals. So it follows that a healthy diet is the opposite: low in unhealthy fats, refined carbohydrates and sugar with few or no food additives, colourings and preservatives, and high in fibre, protein and essential vitamins and minerals. The long-term aim is for you to be eating this type of diet as your 'new normal'.

Eliminate any foods that are processed, refined, preserved or canned. Also eliminate hydrogenated oils (natural oils altered by processing) and any foods containing trans-fats.

Find a local supplier of organic produce and choose organic fruit, vegetables, meat and chicken wherever possible. Organic labelling means that the produce is farmed without pesticides, hormones or growth-promoting agents, and the soil is reconditioned naturally to return nutrients to the soil.

Making sure you eat plenty of vegetables and fruit will ensure adequate fibre intake, which helps the gut to eliminate toxins as well as providing essential nutrition. If you have a sluggish gut or you don't eat plenty of fruit and vegetables, you may need to add a fibre supplement such as psyllium husks.

Ensure you have a daily supply of vitamin C–rich fruit and vegetables, and include plenty of leafy green vegetables such as kale and cabbage; dark red/purple fruit and vegetables such as beetroot and berries; whole grains including brown rice, quinoa and amaranth; raw nuts and seeds, legumes and beans.

Chlorophyll or chlorella in green leafy vegetables or in supplements increases the excretion of fat-soluble toxins. Simple dietary additions such as including more green tea and ginger are also easy ways to support your ongoing detoxification.

Use fresh leeks, onion, garlic and ginger, and turmeric and rosemary in your cooking, and drink 2–3 litres of filtered water, including green tea, each day.

Looking through this list, you may find you see things on trips to your fruit and vegetable supplier or produce market that you have never noticed before, or never thought of buying. You can use the detox phase to experiment with some new food ingredients, tastes and textures.

You might need to scour your recipe books to look for ways of incorporating new ingredients into your home cooking.

THE CAFFEINE QUESTION

Okay, now I know this is a tough one for many of us, but if you are going to be a bit serious about a detox, you do need to look at how much caffeine you drink and eat. You find caffeine in coffee, tea, chocolate, cola drinks, energy drinks and some medications. A couple of cups of coffee a day is fine, but for a detox it is worthwhile reducing your caffeine intake to zero for a few weeks. It can be harsh on your body if you stop caffeine abruptly because the withdrawal from caffeine can cause headaches and make you feel tired and flat for several days.

The more coffee you drink, the more gradually you will need to wean yourself off it. Rather than going cold turkey, start by reducing your total daily intake by one, then after four or five days reduce again until you get to zero. After a few weeks, if you start back on caffeine drinks, try to keep your daily quantities low, at a level where you are unlikely to experience withdrawal effects if you stop it.

ALCOHOL

Alcohol is a legal and socially acceptable drug in moderation. The problem is that not everyone drinks in moderation, not everyone can cope with even 'safe' levels of alcohol, and not all livers are able to process alcohol to the same extent as others. In addition, every liver needs a regular rest, such as two days straight every week, to recover its function.

Some medications stress your liver and can increase your levels of liver enzymes, called 'transaminases'. If you combine those medications with alcohol, then the stress effect on your liver can increase.

If your liver transaminases – liver enzymes released by damaged liver cells – are elevated on a blood test and you do not have a form of viral hepatitis, it is a signal that your liver is not coping with the load of toxins, whether from medications, alcohol or other chemicals.

If you are a habitually heavy drinker, talk to your doctor about an injection of vitamin B (particularly thiamine and folate) to avoid alcohol withdrawal effects. Your doctor will help you assess whether intensive medical intervention is necessary to help you safely withdraw from heavy drinking.

Because the liver is one of the key organs responsible for detoxifying your body, giving it a rest from alcohol will be a key part of any detox program. During the detox phase, avoid alcohol completely for at least a month, longer if your liver function tests are abnormal, or until liver function tests return to normal levels. After that you can make a decision about what level of alcohol you want to resume, ranging from keeping it at zero, and hopefully only increasing it up to the generally agreed 'safe' maximum level of no more than two standard drinks in a 24-hour period, no more than five days a week. (See chapter 'Alcohol' on page 67.)

ILLICIT DRUGS

Illicit recreational drugs are not often disclosed in a medical history, but doctors know their use is common. They can also have a profound long-term effect on your mood and mental functioning and, obviously, are best avoided.

As part of your detox process, any illicit drugs need to be excluded. (See chapter 'Illicit drugs' on page 104.)

MERCURY FILLINGS

Some people have old mercury amalgam fillings removed as part of a detoxification process. Most dentists would advise you to leave stable amalgam fillings in place, and replace them with non-mercury fillings only if you have a problem with that tooth. I don't necessarily agree. There is a very active global campaign underway to eliminate mercury from dentistry altogether. You can make a decision about whether you want to have your mercury amalgam fillings removed.

If you are having a mercury filling removed, it should be done very carefully with special precautions, such as the use of a dental dam, water cooling and strong suction to remove mercury vapours and minimise exposure to mercury particles. You need to discuss the technique with your dentist in advance to make sure they have the right equipment and that they take this seriously.

I would also advise you not to have any new mercury amalgam fillings. Ever. Fortunately this practice seems to be rapidly disappearing from modern dentistry.

TOXINS IN YOUR WORKPLACE

Depending on your industry or occupation, there will be toxins in your workplace. While it will be possible to eliminate some of these, others are an inherent part of the job. If you have an Occupational Health and Safety committee or officer, then it may be possible to raise some issues with them. Obviously if there is protective clothing or breathing apparatus you will be using them. Sometimes simple solutions can be found to reduce your exposure, such as improving ventilation or having air-conditioners serviced regularly, or choosing less toxic cleaning products.

SUPPLEMENTS TO SUPPORT THE DETOX PHASE

A number of herbs and vitamin supplements can assist the detox process, but I would urge you not to self-prescribe. Rather, ask for expert professional advice first.

- **St Mary's thistle** – *or 'milk thistle', is one of the herbs commonly used to support the liver during detox. The active liver-protective ingredient in St Mary's thistle is silymarin, obtained from the seeds. Silymarin is a group of flavonoids (silibinin, silidianin, and silicristin), which are thought to help protect liver cells and repair liver cells damaged by toxic substances.*

- **probiotics** – *increase the 'good bugs' or 'healthy' bacteria in your gut, while reducing the load of 'bad bugs'. A healthy balance of gut bacteria helps with digestion and improves the elimination of some toxins.*

- **iodine** – *check your iodine level with a simple urine test, which your doctor can arrange for you. Iodine deficiency is common, especially on a low salt diet, but it is essential for protecting your immune system and helps to eliminate toxins such as fluoride, bromide and some heavy metals. It is also essential for normal thyroid function.*

- **chlorophyll or chlorella** – *increases the excretion of fat-soluble toxins. It can be supplemented or found in high amounts in green, leafy vegetables and algae.*
- **dietary fibre and fibre supplements** – *rice bran fibre, brown rice and psyllium have been shown to be very effective toxin binders. Make sure you are drinking plenty of water when you are taking extra fibre.*

EXERCISE

Exercise is an essential element of any detox process, just as it is essential for your general health and wellbeing all of the time. Exercise stimulates your circulation and lymphatic system and, indeed, all body processes that help to rid your body of toxins through your excretory organs. It also helps to mobilise fat-soluble toxins.

Make sure you don't overdo it at first, especially if you are suffering any withdrawal effects from alcohol, caffeine or illicit drugs. Gentle exercise such as walking, light yoga, stretching and tai chi are fine no matter what type of detox you choose to do. You can increase the time and intensity of your exercise as your energy levels improve.

The amount of exercise that is right for you during a detox is a very individual thing. Listen to your body and pace yourself.

SLEEP

Getting enough sleep, on a regular basis, helps to give your body time to repair and regenerate. During a detox process, aim for seven to eight hours' uninterrupted sleep every night. (See the chapter 'Sleep' on page 116.)

DETOX YOUR MIND

Stress is an internal toxin that generates potentially harmful chemical by-products in your body. Negative emotions affect your mood and also change your body's physiology through hormones, brain chemicals and the functioning of your immune system.

To reduce the impact of stress and negative emotional states, your detox program will need to include some stress-busting moves such as simple relaxation and breathing exercises, meditation, tai chi or yoga (see chapter

'Stress and mental health' on page 90). You may find that you unearth the need for individual counselling or joining a support group, or decide to make some major decisions about changing the way you live and work.

In the chapter 'Stress and mental health', on page 90, I go into detail about the effects of stress on your moods and physical health, and ways to manage life's pressures.

HEAVY METALS

If you have had medical tests to confirm heavy metal excess in your body, then you will need to see a doctor who specialises in techniques for eliminating these particular toxins. Heavy metal detoxing methods might involve simply eliminating the source of the heavy metal exposure, where that is possible, and using the detox process to give your body the chance to eliminate the toxins as much as possible using your body's own processes of excretion.

Chelation therapy is used by some specially trained doctors to treat heavy metal poisoning, but it is a controversial procedure. Chelation can treat heavy metal poisoning from mercury, lead, iron or copper, but the chelation compounds used during detoxification are potentially toxic themselves and they chelate other essential minerals your body needs to retain, such as calcium and zinc. You will need to carefully weigh up the potential risks and benefits of this therapy.

WHO SHOULD NOT DETOX?

Eliminating, or at least minimising, toxins from your life is a good idea for pretty much everyone. If you are planning a more elaborate or extensive detox process, or you are considering adding herbs or supplements or having intravenous megavitamins, then you will need specialised medical advice. If you are pregnant, breastfeeding, very underweight or have a diagnosed medical condition, then you definitely need to ask for medical advice and supervision.

HOW LONG CAN I EXPECT TO DETOX?

I have had patients and friends who, on my advice, stopped drinking alcohol or smoking and complained to me after two days that they didn't feel any better. In fact, there is every chance you might feel worse for a while before you start feeling better. This is especially the case with withdrawal from caffeine, cigarettes or other drugs with features of dependence or addiction. Some withdrawal effects are the result of toxins being mobilised from body tissues and metabolised. The common symptoms of withdrawal can include headaches, nausea, altered bowel function, dizziness, irritability, anxiety and fatigue. This passes.

A thorough detox can take from two weeks to several months depending on your state of health and your toxin load, and the degree of difficulty you have in eliminating toxins from your life or making substantial changes to your routines and habits. If you have a high toxin load and you need to make a lot of changes, then the detox will take longer. Your timeline needs to be individualised, and you may need professional advice to develop an effective plan for the type and duration of your personal detox program.

RESTORING BALANCE

The duration of a detox depends on your current toxin load and what type of individual detox program you are planning. Every part of your daily life involves a risk of exposure to chemicals, many of which are potentially harmful to health. At the very least, a detox process serves as a consciousness-raising exercise to show you how many ways you are exposed to toxins. Yet many of these toxins can be easily eliminated or replaced with safer habits or alternatives. Part of your strategy to elevate your health to its best level is to identify the toxins you are able to remove from your life permanently and reduce your overall toxin load. This is not just an occasional, once a year fad; living a low-toxin life can be the plan for your long-term future. Your new normal.

Once you have completed the cleansing process, you can decide what you want to reintroduce. For example, you might resume a lower level of drinking alcohol than before, but decide you will not take up smoking again.

We will deal with the long-term planning in the sustain stage.

THE DETOX PHASES

- *See your GP for a comprehensive medical history and examination, appropriate investigation, accurate diagnosis and medical advice.*

- *Do a personal toxin audit of your home, workplace and other environments you visit frequently.*
- *Assess what you will eliminate from your lifestyle and what you will add in*
- *Do a household clean-out*
- *Plan your exercise program*
- *Decide on your relaxation components*
- *Work out a long term strategy for a 'new normal' that you can sustain.*

Reboot your lifestyle

YOUR REBOOT APPROACH

In the coming chapters dealing with your lifestyle, I will ask you to set some goals for yourself along the way to your long-term plan for the sustain phase. Ideal goals for health are based on all the information we have about the links between your health behaviours, your lifestyle habits, the environment and many other influences. There might be a bit of a gap between the ideal and what you feel is realistic for you at a particular time in your life.

Now think about what you believe you can realistically achieve, at least in the first round. Depending on your personality and your current situation, you might approach the reboot in a number of different ways. I see a variety of patterns, all of which can lead to eventual success.

'BOOTS AND ALL'

The 'boots and all' approach will suit if you all of the conditions are right. You might go for this style if the implications of you not making substantial and permanent changes are serious or potentially life-threatening. This might be the case if you have been diagnosed with a serious disease such as cancer or diabetes, or you have had a heart attack. In these situations, the stakes are high and the risks of not making immediate and substantial changes are obvious.

ONE STEP AT A TIME

If a total life renovation feels like too much to cope with all at once, you can take it one step at a time. This can be the situation, for example, with a heavy drinker or a heavy smoker where changing everything all at once could feel like too high a mountain to climb. Start by setting your priorities. You can decide for yourself the most important priority, or discuss it with your doctor or other health adviser. You can set less ambitious initial goals for the next order issues. Once you feel you have that top priority issue under control, you can then incrementally adjust the other priorities.

ALCOHOL

It's as Australian as kangaroos and a day at the footy to 'like a drink'. The problem is that too many Australians are liking alcohol way too much, to the point where it has become one of the top 20 leading causes of disease and injury, making it a major and increasing public health issue.

You might be surprised at the results in your Health Audit about how much you drink. Many of my patients are shocked when we tally up the number of drinks and compare it with what is considered safe for them. In this chapter we will put your drinking habits into the context of what is considered 'safe' and what possible harm you are doing to yourself, and then look at ways to reduce that harm.

I've heard it said that the medical definition of a problem drinker is someone who drinks more than their doctor. In my case, that would make for a lot of problem drinkers. But seriously, I am constantly amazed at how much alcohol is considered 'normal' in some social groups.

Some people consider a bottle or two of wine *per person* in an evening as average. Drink serving sizes are often more than one standard drink so when I point out that the safe maximum is less than a *quarter* of a bottle per person … well, you can imagine the surprise.

To stay within the currently recommended daily limit of two standard drinks, we are talking about a maximum of one-quarter of a bottle of wine – two glasses – in a 24-hour period, no more than five days a week. That's right. A bottle of wine contains an average of around eight standard drinks, so if you share one bottle of wine between two people, which is a common practice, then that is 100 per cent over the safe recommended limit. Double, in fact.

The current recommendation is for a maximum of one or two standard drinks a day, no more than five days a week. And this is likely to continue to be adjusted downwards.

The recommendation for pregnant women is zero.

LOW-RISK DRINKERS

You know you are a low-risk drinker:

- *when everyone assumes you are the designated driver*
- *when you can say 'no' after the second glass of wine*

- *when you find it easy to have days or weeks without drinking alcohol at all*
- *if you think sculling competitions are stupid*
- *if you can have fun with friends, whether you are drinking alcohol or not*
- *if your normal pattern of drinking is well within recommended safe limits.*

If you are a low-risk drinker, then good for you. You can proritise other areas of your health and lifestyle. The important thing is to be alert to any change in your drinking towards a riskier pattern.

You can also read on to identify risky patterns in your family, friends and colleagues.

MEDIUM-RISK DRINKERS

Case study

Jen is a 30-something executive. She was frustrated with her diet because she never seemed to be able to lose those last 5 kilos of weight.

'I have tried every single diet there is,' she told me.

We went through her food and exercise diary. They seemed fairly healthy. If it was all true, there wasn't too much room to move.

'How about alcohol?' I asked her. 'How much do you drink?'

'Oh, pretty average, I'd say.'

'What would you call average?'

'Nothing on Monday to Wednesday. We usually go out for a drink after work on a Thursday night. Have a few cocktails, a couple of wines over dinner.

'Friday and Saturday night we do a few shots, and about half a bottle of wine. Maybe a beer or two after dinner.'

When we counted up, Jen was binge drinking three nights a week, adding up to a total of 30 drinks in an average week. We not only had an explanation for her difficulty in losing weight, but we also knew why her liver function tests were up a bit, and why she had trouble getting motivated early in the week at work.

BINGE DRINKING

Despite the fact that alcohol is known to be dangerous for a developing brain, at least up until the age of 18 and probably into the mid-twenties, up to one-third of adolescents binge drink, and way too many people do not grow out of the habit. Death from acute alcohol consumption is most common in younger people, aged 15 to 29 years. Alcohol use disorder is becoming more common in middle-aged people.

In common usage, a binge is often considered to be 'drinking to get drunk', but in fact the amount of alcohol that can cause you harm may not be enough to make you feel 'drunk'. The amount of alcohol it takes to cause short-term and long-term damage is much less than you may realise.

On a single occasion of drinking, the risk of alcohol-related injury increases with the amount you consume. For healthy men and women, drinking no more than four standard drinks on a single occasion reduces the risk of alcohol-related injury arising from that occasion. For this reason, a 'binge' is generally considered to be four or more drinks – equal to about half a bottle of wine or four nips of spirits – on one occasion.

Most of us would be familiar with scenes of people staggering along the street, vomiting, getting into fights or having accidents, or being unsafe sexually after drinking too much. This is the glaringly obvious picture of the ugliness and danger of intoxication.

Early in my career I spent many Friday and Saturday nights working in hospital emergency departments when we would have to pump out the stomachs of young people who had been brought in unconscious from binge drinking alcohol. They don't always survive. During the 10 years from 1993 to 2002, an estimated 501 under-aged drinkers died from injury or disease related to risky/high-risk alcohol drinking in Australia.

Even if there is no dramatic evidence of heavy alcohol consumption, regular binge drinking has effects on your brain and nervous system, heart, stomach and gut, immune system and musculoskeletal system. The more you drink, the more likely you are to cause damage.

One of the problems is that so many people have adjusted their idea of 'normal' drinking, and technical 'binge drinking' is being considered 'normal'. Although it might be common, it is not safe.

A common question I am asked is this: 'If two drinks a day, five days a week is safe, then that makes ten drinks a week. So, if I only drink on Saturday night, does that mean I can have 10 drinks on one night a week, have a "blinder" and then not drink for the rest of the week?'

'Actually, no!'

Some of the short-term health problems created by binge drinking include:

- *increased risk of injury due to falls and accidents*
- *poor judgement leading to bad decisions*
- *unsafe sexual activity*
- *loss of valuable personal items*
- *hangovers*
- *headaches*
- *nausea and vomiting*
- *shakiness*
- *memory loss*
- *poor work performance the following day*
- *generalised fatigue*
- *nutritional deficiencies*
- *death related to alcoholic poisoning.*

The amount you drink over a short period of time is one issue. The amount you drink on a regular basis over a long time is another.

So the risky patterns are:

- *episodes of binge drinking*
- *long-term excessive drinking.*

It gets down to this: there are lifetime risks in high-risk drinking, and single-episode risks. If you drink more than the safe limit over the long term, it will have chronic effects on your long-term health. If you drink a lot on a single occasion, then you are at higher risk of illness or injury related to alcohol on that occasion. Of course, you might get away with it many times, but your risk is greater that sooner or later there will be an incident.

MEDIUM-RISK DRINKERS: CUTTING DOWN TO SAFE LEVELS

Changing your drinking patterns can be hard if they are closely entwined with your social activities, and especially so if you are surrounded by people who drink as much as you or more. It really has to be an individual decision of whether you want to protect your health for the future.

Some people use events like 'dry July' or 'New Year's resolution January' to take a month off and reset the dial. I often advise people to blame me and tell their friends they have medical advice to do a detox. This is an excellent circuit breaker to give you time to reboot entrenched patterns.

Sometimes the motivation just isn't there to stop drinking, even for a while, so if you can't manage a 'dry month', try for a 'moist month', which is not as 'wet' as your usual habits. Reducing your intake involves cutting down to safer levels by using a variety of techniques.

Techniques for cutting down

- ♣ Decide to stop drinking on most weekdays.
- ♣ Eat before you drink alcohol.
- ♣ If you are thirsty, drink water first, rather than using alcohol as a thirst-quencher.
- ♣ Sip, don't gulp.
- ♣ Invest in a spirit measure for when you are drinking at home as it can be easy to underestimate the amount of alcohol in a nip. Each nip equals one standard drink.
- ♣ Try substituting at least each second drink with a non-alcoholic drink or water. This reduces the amount of alcohol and also keeps up your hydration.
- ♣ You may need to change your social patterns for a period of time to adjust your patterns.
- ♣ Avoid drinking in 'shouts' or 'rounds' because that locks you into the quantity the group drinks, rather than your own limit.
- ♣ If there are only two of you, order wine by the glass or half-bottle rather than sharing a full bottle.
- ♣ Don't let waiters or hosts top up your drink before your glass is empty. If they do, you cannot count how much you are drinking.
- ♣ If you are a woman of childbearing age and not using effective contraception, assume you could be pregnant and be careful not to binge drink at all.

HIGH-RISK DRINKERS

In a clinical setting, a lot of patients I see have no idea that their level of drinking is potentially harmful and is probably responsible for their non-specific symptoms, such as fatigue, weight gain, indigestion, trouble sleeping, recurrent infections, sexual dysfunction, hair loss, depression or flat mood.

Alcohol-related problems

- health problems
- nutritional deficiencies
- anxiety and depression
- sleeping problems
- accidents
- poor performance at school or work
- financial problems
- relationship conflict
- violence
- legal problems: drink driving, assault

LONG-TERM ALCOHOL EFFECTS

In general practice I often need to have the conversation with a patient who is suffering the effects of too much alcohol, or who will suffer effects if they keep going the way they are. It is not enough to say, 'I don't have a problem', because you can 'drink anyone under the table', like that's a good thing. Knowing your way around a hangover doesn't mean you are protected from damage either. The longer you drink to excess, the more likely it will be for you to develop an alcohol-related health problem.

More and more we are recognising the risks of too much alcohol in the longer term. There are the non-specific effects of chronic low-grade toxicity and withdrawal, but we also see an increased risk of high blood pressure, heart disease and stroke, cirrhosis of the liver, pancreatitis, alcohol dependence, malnutrition and some cancers.

Alcohol is a health problem for both genders.

Approximately 40 per cent of Australian men consume alcohol at levels in excess of current recommendations. This results in problems such as increased car accidents, industrial accidents, violence, several cancers, impotence and infertility. Other longer-term issues include financial pressure, poor work performance, and relationship and family problems.

Recently we have recognised a connection between alcohol and an increase in breast, rectal and liver cancer rates in women, with data suggesting that every drink increases the risk of cancer.

A recent international study of more than 40 countries found Australian women ranked third behind Uganda and New Zealand when it came to suffering the social and personal consequences of excessive alcohol consumption.

ALCOHOL AND NUTRITION

Because of the effect of alcohol on the gut and digestive system, excessive alcohol consumption can lead to some subtle and some more overt nutritional deficiencies. If you keep drinking at unsafe levels, you will need to get professional advice about diet and nutritional supplements to avert the more common nutritional deficiencies associated with alcohol. But just correcting nutritional deficiencies will not mean you can keep drinking at harmful levels without risking other long-term health effects.

The extent of any deficiencies will depend on the quality and quantity of nutrients in your diet, your ability to absorb nutrients through your gut, and the amount of alcohol you drink. If you have any gut problems, you will be less efficient at absorbing nutrients from food, and alcohol itself impairs nutrient absorption.

A dietitian can work out the nutrient quality of your diet. Your doctor can arrange blood tests for some (but not all) nutrient levels. To replace deficiencies with supplements, you will need professional advice on combinations and doses. As a general guide only, the most common alcohol-related nutritional deficiencies you will need to consider include:

- **protein** – *you need to make sure you have adequate dietary protein, and protein supplementation may also be necessary*
- **folate** – *alcohol interferes with the absorption of folate and increases excretion of folate by the kidneys. Diet is also often folate-deficient in heavy drinkers. Increasing dietary folate and supplementation can improve health*
- **B vitamins** – *deficiency of most B vitamins is very common with high alcohol intake due to dietary deficiency, impaired metabolism and decreased storage. Deficiency in the B vitamins (particularly thiamine) can cause brain and nervous system damage*

- **vitamin C** – *this deficiency is very common as alcohol speeds up the excretion of vitamin C in urine*
- **calcium** – *long-term excessive alcohol reduces calcium absorption and metabolism and therefore bone formation. Eventually this leads to osteoporosis*
- **magnesium** – *a very common deficiency with a high intake of alcohol, because of high loss in urine. Deficiency of magnesium may contribute to extreme withdrawal effects – delirium tremens or the DTs and abnormal heart rhythms*
- **zinc** – *this mineral is an essential nutrient in immune function, wound healing and protein metabolism, and is responsible for the sensations of smell and taste. Dietary sources are seafood, meat, grains, beans, nuts and dairy products. Zinc deficiency is more common in vegetarians because phytochemicals called 'phytates' in grains and legumes bind zinc and interfere with its absorption. Zinc supplementation helps to reduce liver damage.*

EFFECTS OF ALCOHOL ON SLEEP

Having a drink in the evening to try to help you sleep will have the reverse effect. While alcohol will help you get to sleep, a few hours later, as the alcohol levels in your blood start to fall, there is a stimulant or wake-up effect. If sleep is an issue for you, then you will need to avoid drinking alcohol within four to six hours of going to bed. The muscle relaxant effects of alcohol will also worsen any problem you have with snoring and sleep apnoea.

ALCOHOL DETOXING

If you know you have been hitting the alcohol too hard, then it is a good time to consider a detox (see the chapter 'Detox' on page 51). But if you usually drink more than four or five drinks a day, then you might expect some withdrawal symptoms when you start the detoxification.

Heavier regular drinkers will need some help with their detox, and I would recommend seeking individual professional advice. It would be wise to discuss a plan of action with your doctor. This is particularly the case if you have significant medical problems, if you are on pharmaceutical medication, or you intend to take a combination of supplements. Your doctor can give you an injection of B vitamins, with thiamine and folate being particularly important to help reduce the effects of stopping heavy alcohol consumption.

As a general guide only, the following supplements may be recommended. If your doctor is trained in nutritional or complementary therapies, then they will also be able to advise you about supplements:

- **a multivitamin** *containing B vitamins, magnesium and zinc – to allow a return to adequate nutrient levels. You may need separate B vitamins – high-dose vitamin B can be given as an intramuscular injection – zinc and magnesium supplementation to provide higher doses until levels are normalised*
- **vitamin C** *– helps to reverse fatty liver common in excess alcohol consumption and increases the body's ability to break down the toxic by-products of alcohol*
- **L-glutamine**, *an amino acid – one of the building blocks of protein, helps to protect the liver and kidneys and also decreases craving for alcohol and sugar*
- **lecithin** *– helps mobilise fats out of the liver*
- **St Mary's thistle** *(Silybum marianum) – a herb with thousands of years of traditional use as a liver tonic, its main active constituent is silymarin. It is very popular in hangover remedies and is known to be a potent antioxidant. St Mary's thistle helps the liver to resist damage from toxins, reduces scar formation in the liver and helps liver cell regeneration*
- **Probiotics**, *or gut bugs – are usually out of balance in people who drink heavily. A supplement containing acidophilus and lactobacillus species will help rebalance the gut's microflora.*

TREATMENT FOR HIGH-RISK DRINKERS

If you are a high-risk drinker, you might need specialised alcohol rehabilitation. This is because the effect of withdrawal on the body can be intolerably uncomfortable and even dangerous, and psychological and behavioural therapy can help reduce the risk of relapsing into old habits.

You might be a high-risk drinker if you:

- *crave alcohol and become irritable if you can't get a drink*
- *cannot stop drinking once you have started*

- *can't remember events or conversations*
- *have had problems with the law related to your drinking*
- *have had difficulty maintaining a relationship*
- *have had trouble keeping a job*
- *drink alone or secretively*
- *have liver damage, nerve damage or significant nutritional deficiencies related to alcohol*
- *suffer withdrawal symptoms when you stop drinking.*

WITHDRAWAL EFFECTS

If you have been drinking more than is healthy for you, you may be able to just stop without suffering any noticeable withdrawal effects. If you pay close attention to the days immediately after you have been drinking, particularly, say, if you have been drinking heavily on weekends, you may notice a variety of withdrawal effects over the following days when you are not drinking, including fatigue, anxiety, depression, clouded thinking, trouble concentrating, irritability and jitteriness. More severe effects might include sweating, headaches, trouble sleeping, nausea, rapid heart rate and tremors.

I remember once speaking to an elderly man who was worried he was developing Parkinson's disease because he had developed a tremor so bad that he couldn't hold a cup of tea without spilling it. On close questioning, his tremor came on in the evenings about 5 pm, lasted a few hours and then abated. Each evening he would have a scotch (heavy-handed pour), then a couple of wines with dinner and a scotch or two watching television in the evening. When he measured the nips of scotch and the half-bottle of wine (they were big wine glasses) he totalled up five to eight standard drinks a day. By the next afternoon he was suffering withdrawal symptoms, including the tremor. The first scotch settled the tremor and off went the vicious cycle again.

We corrected his nutritional deficiencies, loaded him up with vitamin B, reduced his alcohol intake and the tremor went away.

The most severe form of withdrawal is called delirium tremens (DTs), with agitation, confusion, hallucinations and the possibility of seizures. If there is a risk of DTs because of heavy drinking, withdrawal will need to be managed under supervision in a medical setting, usually a hospital.

There are medications, such as disulfiram and acamprosate, which can be prescribed by doctors to help manage alcohol cravings and withdrawal symptoms. But again, close supervision is important so that one potentially addictive substance is not replaced with another.

Regular exercise helps to relieve anxiety and depression, which might be part of your reason for drinking or a consequence of your drinking. Counselling and support groups can help you to figure out why you drink excessively and to stay the course of reducing alcohol intake.

In excess, alcohol is not a benign pleasure. But you may not have to quit drinking totally and permanently to stay healthy, unless you have a problem with dependence or if high-risk drinking would put your long-term health at risk if you take it up again.

You may be ready to hear the message about alcohol and do something about it, or you may need to think about it for a while before you are ready to make changes and drink at safe levels. But you won't achieve ultimate wellbeing until you do.

MOVING FORWARD

Once you have assessed your alcohol intake and decided you need to make changes, work out if you want to do a full detox or take a cut-down approach.

In the sustain section we will talk about finding and sustaining your 'new normal' pattern of living.

During the detox process you might have decided to drink no alcohol for some weeks or months. As you move into the sustain phase you will have the opportunity to work out what is the right level of alcohol for you to drink and still achieve ultimate wellness. Unlike smoking, it does not have to be zero to be healthy, although that might be what you decide.

GOALS

Here are a couple of ideas for goals from me:

- *to stay within safe alcohol drinking limits (maximum 2 standard drinks per day, no more than five days per week)*
- *to avoid binge drinking.*

YOUR GOALS

Goal	Action	Obstacles/solutions	Result
To cut back to safe levels	Four alcohol-free nights per week	I like to wind down with a glass of wine. Try to only have two drinks in a sitting	Successfully reduced my overall drinks per week to under ten

SMOKING

Why is anyone still smoking? It beats me. There cannot be anyone in the developed world who does not know how dangerous smoking is to their health. We know the dreadful statistics: damage to heart, lungs and blood vessels and every other body part. Yet, unbelievably, people still continue to light up.

If you are smoking, you are not going to achieve ultimate wellbeing. There. I've said it. You cannot pump through your body even small doses of the poisons contained in a cigarette and expect to be as healthy as you can be.

THE CASE AGAINST CIGARETTES

The case against cigarettes is open and shut, and all the warnings and public health initiatives are having an effect. Major tobacco-related diseases include cancer (particularly lung cancer), heart and blood vessel disease, stroke and chronic obstructive lung disease. Smoking kills more men than women, and smoking rates are higher among younger age groups and people with a lower level of education.

In Australia, greater awareness of the harmful effects of cigarettes has seen smoking rates among men decline steadily. In 1945, at the end of World War II, 72 per cent of men were smokers. Today, it is under 20 per cent.

By comparison, the number of women smokers rose to a peak of 33 per cent in 1976 and it is now back under 15 per cent.

Although the death rates for male smokers are higher than for females, women are by no means immune. In 2004, 18 per cent of deaths from all causes among men and 10 per cent of deaths from all causes among women were attributable to cigarette smoking.

Adolescent girls who smoke have reduced rates of lung growth, and adult women who smoke have poorer lung function.

Women aged 45 to 74 have more than double the risk of dying if they continue to smoke compared with women who have never smoked. Because the lethal poisons from cigarette smoke travel through every part of the body via the bloodstream, women who smoke are also at increased risk of many other health problems, including cancer of the cervix, cancer of the mouth and throat, heart disease and stroke, osteoporosis and reduced fertility.

Women who smoke have a higher risk of ectopic pregnancy and miscarriage. Smokers are younger at natural menopause than non-smokers and may experience more menopausal symptoms.

In pregnant women the health risk is also shared by their unborn baby, who is more likely to have retarded growth, resulting in low birth weight. While you might think 'little is cute', underweight babies are at greater risk of infections and ill health. If a mother smokes during and after pregnancy, the risk of sudden infant death syndrome (SIDS) is increased.

WHY DO YOU SMOKE?

If one of my patients is a smoker, I will raise the subject with them. Some are surprised that I can tell they smoke, especially when they have gone to some lengths to avoid telling me. I have a nose like a beagle in an airport when it comes to cigarette smoke on someone's breath or coming from the pores in their skin. Working in general practice, I get some interesting insights into the range of reasons why people continue to smoke against the tide of reasons not to.

ADDICTION

We know that in broad terms, it is the physical addiction to nicotine and the perceived psychological benefits that keep people smoking. So ask yourself the question 'What got me started?' because this is where you first formed the habit and it is where we can begin the process of unwinding that effect.

BELONGING

When you are young there is great pressure to conform to your peer group. This is because of the primitive and essential need we social beings called humans have to 'belong'. For some people, this need to belong will carry over into adulthood, and you will sometimes see clusters of smokers outside office buildings sharing their disdain for the judgemental looks of non-smokers and bonding over their complaints about the increasing restrictions on places where they can smoke.

Perhaps you are one of those people who took up smoking in your critical late teenage years, which most of us remember for social awkwardness, and where 'fitting in' with the peer group can seem like the most important priority in your life. In some cases, taking up smoking was a form of rebellion against the values of your parents, rules, restrictions or simply 'authority'.

'SOCIAL' SMOKING

While we're talking about belonging, let's do away with the myth of a 'social' smoker. There is nothing social about blowing smoke into the air while you stand outside, separated from other people because your emissions are toxic to others. If you define social smoking as the thing you do every so often when you are having a drink with friends who are smokers, that notion has pretty much disappeared as the dwindling number of smokers shuttle outside, leaving the main group indoors.

There is certainly nothing social about inflicting passive smoking on other people in the vicinity.

ROLE MODELLED

Maybe you started smoking because it was the thing you saw your parents and their friends doing, and made a subconscious connection between smoking and being 'mature' and old enough to make your own independent decisions.

UNHEALTHY STRESS RESPONSE

Perhaps you started smoking because someone suggested it might help you get through a stressful time in your life, and once you started, smoking became a way of self-medicating and then addiction set in. We know that smoking is more common in people with a history of mental health issues such as anxiety or depression.

UNHEALTHY WEIGHT CONTROL METHOD

Some young women smoke to suppress their appetite and keep their weight down. Unfortunately, this creates more problems than it solves.

VICTIM OF MARKETING?

If you are old enough, you will remember when tobacco companies were able to openly and legally advertise their products, using the full gamut of marketing techniques to convince you that smoking was the path to a life of glamour, popularity and looking chic. The tobacco companies put huge amounts of money and resources into advertising cigarettes because advertising works. In many countries, tobacco advertising has largely been banned, but there is still exposure to subtle but effective product placement in movies and television programming.

You will notice in other sections in this book that the health information is divided into levels of risk. There is no low or medium risk with smoking. You are just at risk.

Even if you are only an occasional smoker, quitting is an obvious place to start with a lifestyle renovation.

QUITTING

We know that nicotine has a powerful addictive potential. After inhaling the smoke, nicotine enters your bloodstream and travels to your brain within seconds. Here it triggers chemicals in your brain that make you feel momentary pleasure. But then there's the downside. As the nicotine level in your bloodstream rapidly drops, so does your mood. That's when you light up again. Once you are addicted, overcoming the physical or psychological need to smoke is the challenge.

If you are highly motivated to quit or if you are not strongly addicted, you may find quitting is as easy as just deciding not to light up again. And while quitting can be easy for some people, my observations tell me that for most regular smokers the process can be quite a lot more difficult and complicated.

STOPPING SOCIAL SMOKING

One study of US college students found that social smokers – people who smoke mainly with others rather than alone – smoked fewer cigarettes less often than regular smokers, had lower nicotine dependence, less intention to quit and fewer recent quit attempts than regular smokers. What was most interesting to me, however, was that this study showed that social smoking in young people was a stage on the way to becoming a regular smoker.

If you think of yourself as an occasional or social smoker and you want to improve your health or prevent yourself becoming a regular smoker, then my advice is to quit sooner rather than later, while you are less likely to be addicted. One suggestion I give to my patients is to think about the reason why they smoke socially, and try to do all the things associated with their smoking, but without smoking. So, for example, go out for drinks after work or accept invitations to parties, have a couple of drinks and see your friends, but just don't light up. Make yourself a cup of tea after work so you can unwind but without the cigarette.

There are some people who try this but find it doesn't work for them. Old established patterns can reassert themselves and the activity they enjoy is too closely entwined with the stimulus to light up. Having a few drinks reduces resolve and resistance and it is easy to think, 'Just one or two won't hurt. I can quit tomorrow.'

So I need to use a variety of techniques to help social smokers quit depending on what is likely to work. It might take a few attempts.

The main thing you need to do is to decide how crucial the smoking is to your social life. If you are part of a group where almost all your close friends smoke, then you will need stronger motivation than someone who is the smoking 'odd man out' in a group of mostly non-smokers.

As with people trying to change their alcohol drinking patterns, I offer to take the blame. Seriously. I tell patients they can tell their friends their doctor has told them they had to quit for the sake of their health. You may need to change the way you socialise for a while and spend more time with your non-smoking friends until you are confident you can resist the temptation. Whatever method you use, it has to be your idea and you need to be ready and resolved to change.

HOW TO STOP IF YOU ARE A REGULAR SMOKER

First comes the reason you want to quit. For this you need to consider your motivation. Ask yourself, 'Why do I want to change this behaviour?' Here are some suggestions – see if one of them fits you:

- *I don't want to die young*

- *If I don't die young, I don't want to look older than I am*
- *I don't want to face a battle with cancer or heart disease if I can do something to avoid it*
- *I don't want to lose fitness*
- *My father had a stroke and I don't want to go the same way*
- *I don't want my breath to smell like an ashtray*
- *I am sick of feeling unwell*
- *Inhaling over 80 dangerous chemicals into my lungs just doesn't make sense any more*
- *I am sick of contributing to tobacco company profits. I have better things to do with my money*
- *I want to get pregnant*
- *My children want me to quit because they hear the health messages and don't want me to die.*

Having a reason to quit that makes sense to you is the start. Then comes having the willpower to overcome such a powerful addiction.

Timing is important, too. I tend to be silently impatient, wanting people to simply stop smoking because it is so obviously in their best interest. But I am also realistic enough to know that if the timing is wrong, then quitting is less likely to be successful.

For example, if you are under a lot of emotional stress and you tend to treat smoking as a 'stress reliever', then it would be better to set a date when the stress is lower. Similarly, if you know you get very irritable and have trouble concentrating when you are quitting, pick a time when you have fewer demands, such as a holiday away from work.

If you are making the decision to quit, be aware that different methods work for different people. You might need to try a number of techniques before you find something that is likely to work for you.

You also need to identify and overcome any personal resistance. Over the years I have heard just about every excuse in the book for not quitting, some of them more genuine than others. One that sticks in my memory is the man who told me, 'If my wife didn't hear me coughing and wheezing in the night, she'd worry I was dead.'

Think of your excuses for not quitting, and then ask yourself 'Is this a valid reason or just an excuse?' and 'Is there a method to overcome this excuse?'

I have heard the arguments from smokers that unless you have tried to quit 'cold turkey', you don't know how hard it can be, but I still think it is the best way to go if you can. The discomfort of going cold turkey is worse for some people than for others, and some people do not notice any ill effects at all.

The common withdrawal symptoms are impatience, irritability, anger outbursts, anxiety, depression, difficulty concentrating, insomnia and restlessness. And they can last for up to four weeks, so it is worth warning your nearest and dearest.

Cognitive behavioural techniques, hypnotherapy and meditation techniques will all help. Anecdotally, some people say that acupuncture helped them with the cravings, but evidence does not support this.

The herb St John's wort can help to stabilise your mood and can be started several weeks before your quit date to prepare you for the transition. (Consult your health care practitioner regarding the dosage.) Also let your closest people know you are trying to quit and enlist their support.

Some people will put on weight when they quit smoking. A 3 to 4 kilo weight gain in the months after you quit is common but not inevitable. You will need to plan a comprehensive strategy involving careful attention to what you are eating and start or continue daily exercise.

If you have a history of depression, you will need to have the support of your GP, psychologist or psychiatrist through the process, as depression might become temporarily worse in the early days after you quit smoking.

Tips for quitting cold turkey

- ❧ Cognitive behavioural techniques
- ❧ Hypnotherapy
- ❧ Meditation
- ❧ Relaxation and stress management techniques
- ❧ Acupuncture
- ❧ Recruit support of family, friends or health professionals
- ❧ Healthy diet
- ❧ Daily exercise
- ❧ St John's wort

Case study

Mia began smoking at the age of 17 when she was still at school.

'I started smoking because it was the cool thing to do. Both of my parents were smokers too. By the time I was 37 or 38, smoking had become very socially undesirable. I was smoking 20 or 30 a day.

'I remember when you could still smoke in restaurants and we were out with a group of friends and I lit up at the table. The woman at the table next to ours put up an umbrella to block my smoke, and told me she didn't like my smoke in her face while she was eating. At first I thought she was a bit over the top and I laughed about it, but it made me think. A few weeks later I got up one morning and started coughing, and I coughed up a little bit of blood. I thought, "That's it", and never smoked again. I didn't have any withdrawal symptoms, but I was doing transcendental meditation at the time so that might be why.'

❧ QUITTING GRADUALLY

If stopping suddenly is too difficult, then another way to quit is to gradually reduce the number of cigarettes by stretching out the intervals between one cigarette and the next. When the number per day gets down to about four or five, only light up if you are suffering withdrawal effects and smoke only half that cigarette. Gradually reduce to zero.

❧ NICOTINE REPLACEMENT

I am not a big fan of nicotine replacement therapy (NRT), which is available in the form of patches, gum and inhalers. The problem is that the nicotine in the NRT is still addictive and I have seen a lot of patients still chewing away on nicotine gum many years after they stopped smoking.

One US study published in the journal *Tobacco Control* questioned a group of people who had quit smoking and found that around one-third relapsed every few years. The group using NRT patches and gum were no less likely to relapse than those who had relied on willpower or other methods. Having said that, NRT does seem to help those people who initially have problems with withdrawal symptoms.

If you decide to go with NRT, you will need to view it as a transitional method of weaning yourself off the habit of smoking as well as the addictive effect of nicotine, and you will need a strategy for the gradual reduction of the NRT doses. So, it is better, if you can, to try methods of helping you quit that don't use nicotine.

Case study

Debbie was 40 when she decided to quit smoking.

'I had been smoking a pack a day for about 20 years. I had quit before but started up again because lots of the people I hung out with were smokers. I started using the nicotine patches. I would put on a patch, go out with a group, have about 10 drinks and then forget I had put the patch on and start smoking. [This practice of smoking while you are wearing an NRT patch is called 'turbocharging'.]

'Then the room would start spinning and I would feel sick.

'I decided to stay away from smokers for about three months to remove the temptation to light up. I gradually weaned myself down to the lower dose patches and then stopped using them. Once I hadn't been smoking for a while and my sense of smell returned, I noticed when smokers left a restaurant for a cigarette and then returned, they smelled disgusting. That's when I knew I wouldn't smoke again.'

That was 17 years ago.

☘ OTHER PHARMACEUTICAL 'SOLUTIONS'

I am also sceptical of the hype around pharmaceutical drugs like varencycline for quitting smoking. This medication can have serious side effects, such as cardiovascular events and suicidal thoughts, so you would need to weigh up the risks and benefits.

☘ THE KEY TO SUCCESSFUL QUITTING

The key to successful quitting is to change the patterns and routines you associate with smoking.

Case study

David, a 47-year-old businessman in a high-pressure industry, had developed his own way of winding down at the end of the day. When he got home he would make a cup of tea and sit quietly on his back verandah looking at the garden while he smoked a couple of cigarettes. He had developed high blood pressure and because his father had had a heart attack in his fifties, we talked about how important it was for him to stop smoking.

He was reluctant to give up his evening ritual, so I suggested trying the cup of tea and the quiet interlude on the back verandah but leaving out the cigarette. He replaced it with yoga-style deep breathing exercises. David came back to have his blood pressure checked a month later. The change had worked. He still got to wind down after a big day, and realised he didn't need cigarettes to be able to do it.

Take a whole-lifestyle approach

- *Take up a fitness routine or increase your current physical activity level.*
- *Eat a healthy low-fat diet.*
- *Learn new ways of managing stress.*
- *Avoid friends and family who smoke.*
- *Avoid situations/occasions where you habitually smoke.*
- *If you smoke when you drink, consider cutting out alcohol for a few weeks.*
- *Take up a pleasurable activity/hobby that fills the gap.*

Think about how you think about smoking

Your mindset will have a big influence on how successful you are in quitting. A lot of people see cigarettes as their little friends who help make them feel more confident, or more relaxed. Some say they 'love' smoking. If that sounds like you, then you need to see the cigarette as the enemy rather than companion or part of your identity. Focus on the reality of smoking: smelly breath, wheezy cough, yellowed teeth, bouts of bronchitis, deep wrinkles across your face, so puffed you can't walk from one room to another without stopping to catch your breath. Look at your children, your partner, your friends and think of them losing you to a smoking-related disease.

Then believe that you can be a healthier version of yourself if you just give your body a chance to be permanently cleansed of the cocktail of chemicals in every cigarette.

❧ HOW LONG BEFORE YOU BENEFIT FROM QUITTING?

According to the American Cancer Society:

- **20 minutes after quitting** *your heart rate and blood pressure drop*
- **12 hours after quitting** *the carbon monoxide level in your blood drops to normal*
- **2 weeks to 3 months after quitting** *your circulation improves and your lung function increases*
- **1 to 9 months after quitting** *coughing and shortness of breath decrease; cilia, the tiny hair-like structures that move mucus out of the lungs, start to regain normal function, increasing your ability to handle mucus, clean the lungs, and reduce the risk of infection*
- **1 year after quitting** *your excess risk of coronary heart disease is half that of a continuing smoker's*
- **5 years after quitting** *risk of cancer of the mouth, throat, oesophagus and bladder are cut in half. Cervical cancer risk falls to that of a non-smoker. Stroke risk can fall to that of a non-smoker after 2–5 years*
- **10 years after quitting** *your risk of dying from lung cancer is about half that of a person who is still smoking. The risk of cancer of the larynx, the voice box and pancreas decreases*
- **15 years after quitting**: *your risk of coronary heart disease is that of a non-smoker's.*

MOVING FORWARD

YOUR GOALS

Goal	Action	Obstacles/solutions	Result
To quit smoking	Cut back gradually	Lots of my friends are social smokers: spend some time with non-smoking friends	Successfully cut down. On the way to quitting

STRESS AND MENTAL HEALTH

The term 'stress' is thrown around a lot these days. Where once the standard greeting might have been, 'Lovely weather, isn't it?' these days you are more likely to hear 'Hi, been busy?' I guess this is an acknowledgement of the high expectations many of us have of ourselves to manage our homes, families, jobs, hobbies and interests.

Whether you perceive something to be stressful depends on your perspective and your ability to cope with the pressure of your commitments, responsibilities or relationships. Chances are if there is unmanaged stress or situations you are not able to cope with in your life, you will be falling far short of the best your health can be. Left unchecked, stress can become a problem for your emotional and physical health, with far-reaching repercussions.

So many patients I see in general practice are suffering from the effects of what we would commonly call 'stress'. Their symptoms are entirely due to the consequences of unmanaged pressure or emotional overload, or stress is contributing to their level of ill health. On the flip side, being unwell can make it difficult to cope with life's demands, and this also contributes to your sense of stress.

The mind and body are not separate entities; they are parts of the whole and entirely interconnected. If your stress responses are activated over the long term, then you will inevitably suffer consequences to your psychological wellbeing, which can ultimately lead to a clinical diagnosis of depression or anxiety disorder. The solution does not lie in a bottle of booze or a packet of pills, although if the situation becomes severe, medication may be necessary for relief of your symptoms.

Stress affects not only your emotional health but can also have a profound effect on your physical wellbeing, causing physiological wear and tear. Prolonged stress can lead to impaired immunity, increased blood pressure, acceleration of cardiovascular disease, premature ageing – do I have your attention now? – and numerous other medical conditions.

Chances are that if you recognise the early signs of stress, then there is a lot you can do to change your circumstances and improve your mood and your overall wellbeing.

CAN STRESS HAVE BENEFITS?

There is no question that too much stress, or at least too much unmanaged stress, is a bad thing for you. But can stress have some benefits? Absolutely! The pressure involved with preparing for a performance or a work project or for an exam helps you to increase your productivity, find your limits and extend your abilities.

An acute stress response is usually called the 'fight or flight response'. It is the body's surge of chemicals and immune cells in response to an emergency situation, such as an immediate threat to your safety. An example would be the sudden burst of energy, increased heart rate and reflexes and sharpened mind that comes if you need to suddenly act to avoid a car accident.

Short bursts of stress also prime your immune system to deal with infections. But excessive stress over longer periods of time increases your immune system's activity and eventually depletes your resources. This can worsen any inflammatory conditions and ultimately impair the functioning of your immune system.

MANAGING PRESSURE

The aim therefore is not to completely avoid pressure or stress but to find a balance so that pressure is a positive factor in your work and personal life, and does not tip over into chronic, unrelenting pressure where you never get to feel as though you are on top of things or can get away from worries.

What can we do about the negative effects of stress?

When it comes to talking about ways of coping with the pressures of life, a lot of the following advice will sound like plain common sense. But there is great value to be had in a not-so-gentle nudge to remind us of what is really important, rather than allowing ourselves to get bogged down and overwhelmed by commitments and problems at home and at work. I advise you to take an approach that has a multiple focus. By this I mean that you need to look at:

- *treating the consequences of stress*
- *arranging your life so that pressures are manageable*
- *putting in place prevention strategies so that you recognise the early signs of burnout and take action.*

Ask yourself the hard questions:

- *Am I happy at home or are there problems that need to be sorted out?*
- *Am I in the right job?*
- *Are there activities in my life that steal time without being of value?*
- *Am I doing all I can to maintain my physical health?*
- *Have I fallen into any unhealthy habits to help me cope with stress?*

Go to the Health Audit on page 15 and answer the questions about your emotional health and wellbeing.

Once you have honestly answered these questions, you can move on to looking at ways of getting more out of life. Work out what is causing you stress and eliminate or change it. Some changes you can manage yourself, while other changes will need the cooperation of work colleagues, close friends or professional advisors.

✿ TRIAGE

In medical emergency situations there is a system for prioritising the level of response, which is based on the seriousness of the situation. This concept had its origins on the battlefield, where there were basically three categories of casualties: those who will survive whether they get medical care or not; those who will die whether they get medical care or not; and those whose outcome will be improved by getting immediate attention. The medical teams focus their limited resources on the last group, where immediate intervention will make a difference to the patient's outcome.

In your daily life, if you are under pressure and not managing the stress well, you are thinking, and your body is reacting, as if everything is a high-level emergency. What you need to do is develop a personal system of triage.

Think about the situation that is causing you stress. Is there likely to be a serious life-threatening or life-changing consequence if you don't react as if this is an acute emergency? Is this a situation that can go on the backburner for a few hours, days or weeks ... or forever ... with little impact on the outcome? In short, is your response in proportion to the threat?

The other thing that medical teams do is to call for help. If they get word there is a major trauma coming into the emergency unit, they page the team and they come running.

If you have a major issue going on in your life, do you call for help? Do you delegate or outsource some of the tasks you don't actually need to do yourself? Or do you try to do everything and wind up exhausted and overwhelmed?

It is so easy to allow yourself to get swamped with the little things that you can lose sight of the big picture. Rank your 'to do' list from the most urgent to the trivial. Learn to say no to things that are not important if you do not have the time for the important things.

Your triage questions

* Is this situation a bona fide emergency?
* Will this problem matter in a year or two?
* Is this a battle I need to take on right now?
* Is this my problem or someone else's responsibility?
* What is the most important task right now?
* What do I have to do, or what help do I need, to get this task done?
* Is the timeframe I have set realistic for what needs to be accomplished?

ORGANISE YOURSELF

Spend some time each evening planning the next day and the coming week. Mark each task or event with a priority rating (high, medium, low).

Check your high-priority list and make sure all of those items get enough time set aside in your diary. Anything that is less urgent and can wait should wait.

Look at your work practices and see where you can be more efficient or share the workload when the pressure is on. Ask for assistance or delegate tasks that can be done by others if you are short of time. Schedule the most difficult tasks of each day for times when you are fresh, such as first thing in the morning.

GET MOVING

Practically any form of exercise helps you manage stress. Exercise elevates your mood and relieves symptoms of anxiety and depression, and reduces levels of the body's stress hormones, such as adrenaline and cortisol. It also helps improve the quality of your sleep. Higher intensity exercise increases your brain's production of endorphins, the natural neurotransmitters that elevate mood. Improved fitness will help you achieve your goals.

Planning to exercise with a friend can be a regular social connection as well as an incentive to do the exercise on days when it is tempting to stay in bed or skip the activity part of your day plan.

Whatever your age or state of fitness, there is a form of exercise that will improve your wellbeing. It's just a matter of finding it. You might combine a variety of different exercise types so you have a range of intensities. For stress reduction, 45 to 60 minutes a day, five to six days a week is ideal. If you have a health problem that limits your activity options, arrange a session with an exercise physiologist so you can work out an exercise program to suit your abilities.

Make exercise a regular diary entry like any other important meeting or appointment. Look at your schedule and see how you can fit it in. And remember that there are lots of opportunities to 'get moving' during the day. Take the stairs instead of the elevator, walk the children to school instead of driving, take your walking shoes to work and go for a stroll at lunchtime.

❧ YOU ARE WHAT YOU EAT

You will not perform at your best in any part of your life if you are short of essential nutrients, and taking a multivitamin won't make up for a fundamentally poor diet. Day to day, think about everything you eat. When you are stressed, you may lose your appetite in the short term. As the stress becomes chronic, you can tend towards overeating as the stress hormone cortisol stimulates your appetite for high-energy foods. We know that physical or emotional stress increases your intake of foods that are high in fat, or sugar, or both. You may not make time to eat regularly or pay attention to the quality of the food you are eating.

I commonly see people who resort to 'stress snacking', especially in the afternoons if they have not eaten properly early in the day and are looking for a quick 'sugar fix'. Whatever happens, make time for breakfast. Keep your diet low in fat and preservatives and include lots of fresh fruit and vegetables, nuts and grains. Look through the chapter 'Nutrition', on page 132, for a general guideline to healthy eating.

❧ ABUSING SUBSTANCES

Are you smoking 'to cope with stress'? Drinking lots of coffee to combat tiredness? Having a few drinks of alcohol because it helps you wind down or gets you to sleep? Taking sedatives to calm you down or help you get to sleep? Smoking the occasional cannabis to 'chill-ax'? Then you have signs of trouble.

Rather than helping you cope with stress, relying on substances to keep you going just temporarily masks the symptoms. The better approach is to take stock, recognise the sources of stress and deal with them.

❧ STAY ON TOP OF YOUR HEALTH

Do not forget regular health check-ups, even when you are feeling well. I cannot overstate how important it is for you to have your own GP and see them regularly. Ideally, you will see your GP for all the preventive health checks that are recommended for your age, and get on top of any health conditions as soon as they arise.

❧ HOME LIFE

It's very easy to take out your frustrations, anger or distress on the people who are closest to you, so make every effort to avoid doing this. Instead, tell them about your problems and ask for their support and suggestions.

If the problems and stresses are originating from your home and family environment, attempt to talk through the issues to find practical solutions where you can and ask for professional counselling help if necessary.

❧ REMEMBER TO RELAX

If you think you are too busy to find time to relax, then you are not alone. Many people find they actually have to factor leisure time into their diaries, or the time gets eaten up with work and other responsibilities. Think about what you love doing, whether it is reading a good book, going to a concert, having a picnic in the park, and make time for it – ideally, a little every day.

❧ DON'T FORGET TO DREAM

Children dream constantly of what they want to do with their life, what they want to achieve. As we get older we may get wiser but we so easily lose sight of what we really want out of life. This advice may sound like a cliché, but it is never too late to have plans and ambitions for yourself, to decide what is really meaningful to you. Of course your goals have to be realistic, but if you actively set out to make a list of the things you want to achieve, both small and large, you will have a greater chance of success. Concentrate on positive plans for the future, rather than dwelling on what might have been.

❧ TURN DREAMS INTO REALITY

We have business plans for business, game plans for sporting events and financial plans to ensure financial security. Formulating a 'game plan' for the next few years of your life is at least as important. Figure out how you can turn your dreams into reality, step by step, and be prepared to be flexible. If one way doesn't work out, try another.

ACTIVITIES TO HELP YOU MANAGE STRESS

So you have assessed your lifestyle, your work, your home life and your health habits and taken action to address any problems you have identified. Whether or not you decide on seeking professional help, there are some additional activities you can try to help with stress management.

❧ MEDITATION

Possibly the most powerful and effective method of managing stress is to regularly practise meditation. You will find some form of meditation in most of the major religions and spiritual traditions, and meditation is now commonly recommended as an activity that will benefit your health and wellbeing.

There are many different forms of meditation, but most of them have common elements. They generally require:

- *a quiet environment*
- *a comfortable posture, whether sitting, lying or standing*

- *a focus of attention, which may be a mantra, your senses or your breathing*
- *an ability to observe without judgement.*

The aim of meditation is to create a wakeful but relaxed state of mental and physical calm. The most common forms are transcendental meditation and mindfulness meditation.

Transcendental meditation is a part of Ayurvedic tradition. It uses a repeated sound or mantra as the focus of attention. This form of meditation emphasises positive emotions and the need to be in tune with your body's natural rhythms.

Mindfulness practice involves bringing your focus to the here and now. In a nutshell, it involves you giving deliberate and non-judgemental attention to the present moment, where you acknowledge and accept every thought, every feeling and sensation in and around you at that given moment.

If you are planning to practise transcendental meditation or mindfulness mediation, then you will need to be taught by an expert. There is extensive research on the effects of mindfulness practices to show that it is helpful in the treatment of pain, stress, anxiety, eating disorders, addictions, preventing relapse of depression and other situations. We also know meditation changes brain activity, which results in an improvement in mood.

Long-term benefits of meditation

- improved physical health
- enhanced immunity
- improved mental and emotional health
- faster rehabilitation after illness
- clearer thinking
- greater self-awareness
- reduced feelings of stress
- greater resilience to pressure
- improved sense of spiritual fulfilment
- improved quality of life

One study measured electrical activity in the brain before, immediately after, and then four months after an eight-week training program in mindfulness meditation. The results showed significant increases in left-sided frontal brain activation, a pattern known to be associated with positive mood, in meditators compared with non-meditators. The study also found significant increases in the antibody response to influenza vaccine among people in the meditation group.

Long-term meditation is thought to affect not only the electrical activity in the brain but the actual structure of the brain, and to slow age-related loss of brain cells, particularly in brain regions associated with attention and sensory processing. There is also a measurable increase in immune function and changes in other parts of the body.

Meditation can be used to maintain your general wellbeing or as a part of integrative therapy for a range of illnesses. You can also use it to enhance your spiritual development. The physiological and psychological benefits of meditation accumulate over time and with experience.

❧ RELAXATION TRAINING

Yes, believe it or not, you might need to be taught to relax, because relaxing is not always as simple as lying down and closing your eyes. Thoughts and worries can intrude into your consciousness. If you are very stressed, you might find some of your muscles are tense.

Breathe easy

- ❧ Lie down or sit comfortably in a quiet room.
- ❧ Play some peaceful, 'smooth' instrumental music without a defined beat.
- ❧ Close your eyes.
- ❧ Breathe in deeply and slowly through your nose. Do not overfill your lungs.
- ❧ Pause briefly.
- ❧ Breathe out slowly and steadily.
- ❧ Gradually increase the duration of the out-breath so that it is about twice as long as the in-breath.
- ❧ Slow down the breathing cycle, but make sure it feels comfortable and not strained for you.
- ❧ Continue for 10 to 15 minutes.
- ❧ Repeat daily.

The physiological relaxation response slows your heart rate, lowers your blood pressure, and decreases oxygen consumption decreases your levels of stress hormones. There are a number of relaxation techniques you can learn, including slow breathing, progressive muscle relaxation, visualisation and various meditation techniques.

Some of these techniques are taught in yoga schools, private or group classes or in private sessions with a psychologist.

Once you have practised slow breathing, you can use it to restore your balance momentarily at times when you are feeling very stressed. Breathe. Easy.

❧ PROGRESSIVE MUSCLE RELAXATION

This form of relaxation is, as the name suggests, a methodical way of consciously tensing a muscle group and then releasing it, starting at your toes and finishing at your neck and head. It can be taught in groups or private lessons with a psychologist, other healthcare practitioner or yoga teacher, or with a self-help DVD, CD, podcast or app. Once you have been instructed in the technique, you can usually practise it yourself.

❧ AUTOGENIC TRAINING

Autogenic training is a technique that uses both awareness of your body and visual imagery to induce a relaxed state. During autogenic training you may be asked to imagine a peaceful place and then focus on physical sensations such as your pulse or breathing, warmth or heaviness, again moving from your feet to your head.

❧ BIOFEEDBACK

Biofeedback is a technique that helps you learn to control your reactions and some of your body processes using specialised technical equipment to measure your pulse, blood pressure, muscle tension and skin temperature. During biofeedback training you are taught to relax by observing a physiological marker such as your blood pressure or pulse on a monitor and learning how to change it. Eventually you learn to achieve a more relaxed state in any situation, without feedback from the monitors.

COGNITIVE BEHAVIOUR THERAPY

Shows you how to adjust your thinking about yourself and your circumstances and change negative thought patterns and damaging behaviours. In a nutshell, the aim is to gain control of your reactions to stress. This is achieved by teaching you to recognise the thought patterns that produce anxiety and changing your behavioural responses to avoid the anxiety reaction. CBT is most often taught by GPs, counsellors and therapists.

MOVEMENT-BASED THERAPIES

Activities like tai chi, qi gong, yoga and the Alexander technique are primarily movement based. Because they all emphasise focus and awareness, they have a lot in common with meditative practices.

These therapies should all be taught by experts. They can have a range of benefits for psychological issues, including stress as well as physical benefits.

CHANGE WHAT YOU CAN

Do you feel trapped by your circumstances? Perhaps change is well within your reach.

Think of yourself sitting in a cage. You can see out through the bars. You can even reach out, touch, hear and smell your surroundings. The door of the cage is locked. You look down to your clenched fist. Slowly you open your hand. In the palm of your hand lies a key. It is the key to the door of the cage.

What will you do?

Will you sit and look at the key?

Will you hold the key tight, occasionally reaching out through the bars to sample what is 'out there', only to return your arms to the relative safety of your confinement?

Or will you take the key, insert it in the lock, turn it and open the door?

If you open the door, will you step out into the open and see what possibilities lie beyond the immediate distance of your reach or your senses?

So many people are sitting in the cage holding the key to the lock on the cage door. If you are feeling trapped, think of how freedom might look and feel to you.

All the strategies for managing stress are about exploring how your life can be when you free yourself from the things that cause you to feel stressed, overwhelmed, sad, anxious or negative. You may not have the key to all your problems, but you will feel the difference to your life when you change what you can.

HIGHER LEVEL RISK

Stress and anxiety often coexist with depression. Look out for signs that you are slipping into a more precarious mental health state:

- *loss of interest in usually enjoyed activities*
- *insomnia, often with early-morning wakening*
- *reduced appetite*
- *low energy and motivation*
- *little or no interest in sex, if this is unusual for you*
- *. poor memory and concentration*
- *a sense of hopelessness, helplessness and guilt.*

SIGNS OF STRESS

Signs that stress is getting out of control might include:

- *fatigue*
- *headaches*
- *heart palpitations*
- *depression or anxiety*
- *feelings of being overwhelmed and unable to cope*
- *a drop in your work performance*
- *an increase in sick days or absenteeism*
- *trouble sleeping*
- *reduced ability to concentrate or make decisions*
- *gastrointestinal upsets, such as diarrhoea or constipation*
- *using more drugs, alcohol, medications, coffee, chocolate*
- *increased irritability or aggression*
- *deterioration of your personal relationships*
- *increased susceptibility to accidents*
- *poor health, including an increased risk of cardiovascular disease.*

Alcohol and some medications can make you feel depressed, so I would always review any medications you are taking, including indomethacin, griseofulvin, isotretinoin, tetracyclines, beta-blockers and levodopa in case they are responsible for you feeling depressed.

If you are suffering from the effects of anxiety and depression, an integrative approach to improving your mental health is needed. This will mean looking at all the fundamentals of good health, including diet, exercise, sleep, medications, reducing alcohol and substance use, and building your coping strategies and the quality of your relationships.

❧ PROFESSIONAL HELP

Some stress can be solved by assessing your life, thinking about things from different angles and deciding to make positive changes. Talking to your partner, a friend, a mentor or work colleagues can help. But there are times when the best approach is to call for professional help.

You need professional help if:

- *talking to your partner or friends does not help you feel better*
- *you feel sad or anxious most of the time and self-help methods are not working*
- *there is a problem in your life that occupies a lot of your thinking and you cannot see a solution*
- *you start to think of harming yourself or others*
- *your emotional problems or stress are affecting your work or relationships and you cannot identify or solve the problems*
- *there are troubled events in your past that you find hard to talk about.*

To decide which mental health professional is best for your situation, talk to your GP about a referral.

The chapter 'Choosing the Right Health Professionals', on page 34, describes the differences between psychiatrist, psychologist or counsellor. If you are going to see a counsellor, you will need to check out their qualifications and experience, and their areas of special interest and training to see if they are suitable to help you with your problem.

MOVING FORWARD

Here are a few ideas from me about goals you might consider setting for yourself to ensure you have optimal emotional and mental health.

WORK GOALS

- *To ensure that my work is challenging but not overwhelming*
- *To change my work environment or change jobs if I am not happy at work.*

LEISURE ACTIVITIES/HOBBIES GOALS

- *To introduce at least one leisure activity or hobby that I enjoy and can look forward to regularly*
- *To try something new.*

EMOTIONAL WELLBEING GOALS

- *To complete the Kessler Psychological Distress Scale, or K10, to rate my general level of emotional wellbeing (See the Health Audit page 15)*
- *To assess the influences on my emotional world*
- *To seek professional counselling if emotional, relationship or family problems need special attention*
- *To mend broken relationships where possible, or to forgive and move on if not possible.*

YOUR GOALS

Goal	Activity	Obstacles/solutions	Result
To reduce my work stress	Use the 'triage' method to sort out priorities. Breathing exercises	Too much going on all the time: take some extra time to organise myself	Feel better and more relaxed

ILLICIT DRUGS

You might wonder why I am devoting a chapter of a book on ultimate wellness to the subject of illicit drugs. The reason is that illicit drug use is common, but often it is the 'elephant in the room' – the issue that is not discussed unless there is a crisis that needs urgent intervention. A complete audit of all the factors that could be keeping your health in the 'ordinary' category needs to include every possibility, especially given the widespread use of drugs like cannabis and cocaine.

In common usage, the term 'drug' encompasses a large number of substances, including alcohol, prescription medicines and over the counter preparations. Many people use alcohol and tobacco, and some people use illicit drugs. That might be out of curiosity, or because it is something their friends do, or they are looking for a 'buzz' or a new experience.

Illicit drug use needs to be on the agenda because if you use, even just occasionally, it will almost certainly have a negative effect on your wellbeing. Sometimes the effects are massive and obvious. Most often, however, the people I see who are using drugs 'recreationally' as a part of their social life do it in the belief that it is just 'a bit of fun', or 'no worse than a few drinks'. But what they often do not realise is that the effects on their mood and general health can be subtle and gradual.

You know it can't be good for you. To be frank, nobody using illicit drugs can expect any long-term upside. The best you can hope for is no serious damage or mishaps.

If you are thinking, 'It doesn't concern me', then you may need to think again. In Australia, illicit drug use has risen from 13.4 per cent prevalence in the population over 14 years of age in 2007 to 14.7 per cent in 2010, according to the National Drug Strategy Household Survey, and ecstasy and cannabis remain the most commonly used illicit drugs. Even if you don't use illicit drugs yourself, chances are someone close to you does, so it might be handy to be aware of potential problems on behalf of a friend or family member.

I will list a few of the more commonly used drugs to give you an idea of the scope of the issue. Obviously this is not a complete list, but it will give you a picture of some of the consequences of illicit drug use and abuse.

CANNABIS

The most popular illicit drug in Australia is cannabis. The fact that cannabis is illegal while alcohol and tobacco are not is probably more a historical artefact than a reflection of its relative potential danger to personal or public health. Actually, it is so commonly used that a lot of people don't even think of cannabis as 'illicit', even though they know it is illegal.

I know one couple in their fifties who didn't even think to hide a stash when they saw a drug detection dog approaching with a police officer at a music festival and ended up having to defend a charge of possession.

According to the 2010 National Drug Strategy Household Survey, 35.4 per cent of the Australian population reported using cannabis at some time in their lives, with 1.9 million people having used it in the last 12 months. It is estimated that at least 200,000 people are dependent on cannabis in Australia, and one in 10 people who try the drug have problems stopping its use. Obviously, these are sizeable numbers.

There are basically two forms of the drug: marijuana and hashish. Marijuana is made from the dried flowers and leaves, and hashish is made from the resin of the cannabis plant, which is dried and pressed into blocks and smoked or added to food such as cookies and eaten.

Most users smoke cannabis on its own or mixed with tobacco in a hand-rolled cigarette, usually known as a joint. Sometimes it is smoked in a type of pipe called a bong, which cools the smoke before it is inhaled.

There are many active ingredients in cannabis, but the main one is tetrahydro-cannabinol or THC. Extracts in the form of a mouth spray are available in some countries to treat medical conditions such as neuropathic pain in multiple sclerosis patients.

SHORT-TERM EFFECTS

The short-term effects of cannabis include:

- *a feeling of relaxation and loss of inhibitions*
- *bloodshot eyes*
- *increased appetite – 'the munchies'*
- *dry mouth*
- *sleepiness.*

Under the influence of cannabis, a user will get the giggles and feel they have a deeper, more meaningful insight into life but are likely to be talking nonsense. The effect can sometimes be unpleasant with:

- *dizziness*
- *loss of coordination*
- *anxiety*
- *paranoia.*

Cannabis is very risky for people with respiratory conditions, such as bronchitis or asthma, or who have a predisposition to mental illness.

LONG-TERM EFFECTS

If you smoke cannabis then you are at a higher risk of smoking-related diseases such as bronchitis and lung cancer, even if you do not smoke tobacco. Hand-rolled, unfiltered marijuana cigarettes contain up to four times more tar than tobacco.

Longer term, there is a risk of dependence, problems with memory, concentrating and learning, and decreased motivation to work or study.

If you use cannabis to escape from life's problems, the problems do not go away. Prolonged or heavy use of cannabis creates other problems, so the healthier option is to find practical solutions, possibly with the help of a counsellor.

Cannabis can trigger schizophrenia in people who are predisposed to it.

If you are wanting to get pregnant any time soon, you will need to know that cannabis affects a man's sperm count and quality, which can affect fertility. Using cannabis during pregnancy lowers birth weight and increases the likelihood there will be problems for the baby.

QUITTING

If you are a regular cannabis user, you may find you get withdrawal effects when you stop using cannabis, including trouble sleeping, irritability, mood swings, tremors, sweating and abdominal cramps. These effects usually last about two weeks.

Tips to help you quit include:

- *set a date and commit to it*
- *change your lifestyle by avoiding situations where you would usually smoke, at least for the first few months*
- *let your friends know you have quit*
- *find new interests and activities to replace smoking cannabis.*

ECSTASY

Ecstasy is a 'designer' drug related to amphetamines. Its technical name is 3,4-methylenedioxymethamphetamine, or MDMA. It is usually swallowed as a tablet but is also taken in capsules or powder, and is sometimes injected or snorted.

Ecstasy tablets are produced in backyard laboratories, so what people think is MDMA is usually laced with other unknown substances or drugs, and the dosage and quality varies dramatically.

Ecstasy is the second most commonly used illicit drug in Australia. About 10 per cent of the Australian community report that they have tried ecstasy at some time, and about 3 per cent have used it in the past year.

SHORT-TERM EFFECTS

The effects of ecstasy come on after about 30 minutes and last for two to three hours. They include:

- *a state of euphoria or 'ecstasy'*
- *an increased feeling of confidence and lowering of inhibitions*
- *feelings of anger subside and 'everyone loves everyone'*
- *energy level seems to rise*
- *pulse rate and blood pressure rise.*

Some ecstasy experiences are unpleasant. There may be:

- *sweating*
- *severe nausea*
- *jaw clenching and teeth grinding*

- *hallucinations and anxiety*
- *blood pressure and pulse rate increase.*

There are risks to health with the use of ecstasy, and there have been some reports of deaths.

Not much is known about the possible long-term effects of using ecstasy, but it is thought to contribute to depression, memory loss and impaired thinking.

METHAMPHETAMINES

Methamphetamines are completely man-made substances, first developed more than a century ago and used over the years in a number of medical applications, including relieving nasal congestion, assisting weight loss in obesity and treating depression. Amphetamines are classed as stimulants, and are usually taken orally, although some users snort them or inject them into a vein. Because of their stimulant effect, some people use them to stay awake when they are studying, driving long distances or partying all night.

The chemicals used to make 'speed' were made illegal in the late 1980s, so the amphetamines available on the street are usually produced in illegal laboratories.

Amphetamines come in the form of powder, tablets, paste and liquid and have very variable amphetamine content, often containing extra substances that may be dangerous. When they are sold on the street, they are packaged in 'foils' – wrapped in aluminium foil – plastic bags or small balloons. They have a distinctive strong smell and bitter taste.

Some amphetamines, such as dexamphetamine are currently available legally but controversially for the treatment of attention deficit disorder (ADHD) in children and adults. Another medical condition where amphetamines are useful is in the treatment of narcolepsy, which causes a person to suddenly and unexpectedly fall asleep.

SHORT-TERM EFFECTS

The short-term effects of taking amphetamines include:

- *euphoria or a sense of wellbeing and confidence*
- *everything seems to speed up and the user may become talkative, restless and excited*

- *panic attacks*
- *irritability*
- *hostility*
- *sweating*
- *nausea*
- *dry mouth*
- *teeth grinding*
- *increased blood pressure and heart rate*
- *enlargement of the pupils of the eye*
- *headache*
- *reduced appetite.*

Some people use them as an unhealthy method of weight control.

Amphetamines raise body temperature so there can be an added danger if taken with ecstasy.

OVERDOSE

Symptoms of overdose include:

- *chest pains*
- *pounding heart*
- *rapid breathing*
- *panic*
- *shaking*
- *sweating.*

LONG-TERM EFFECTS

Long-term amphetamine use can cause:

- *sleeping disorders*
- *loss of appetite*
- *high blood pressure*
- *irregular heartbeat.*

Heavy users of amphetamines may develop malnutrition if they do not eat properly.

Heavy use of speed can cause brain damage and stroke. If it is injected, impurities in speed can cause abscesses and damage to organs such as the heart, lungs, liver and brain. It is estimated that the content of the average amphetamine produced for illicit supply may be as low as 5 per cent, with the other 95 per cent consisting of impurities.

Used long-term, you can develop withdrawal symptoms when you stop taking it. Withdrawal symptoms can include:

- *hunger*
- *extreme tiredness*
- *depression*
- *anxiety attacks*
- *irritability.*

'SPEED PSYCHOSIS'

This is a temporary state, which is the result of taking too much speed. Features of speed psychosis include:

- *bizarre behaviour*
- *hallucinations – hearing voices and seeing things that are not there*
- *paranoia.*

Some users may become irritable and argumentative or violent.

The symptoms usually go away after a period of not using the drug, but sometimes other medication may be needed to counter the effects.

COCAINE

Cocaine is a stimulant that speeds up the activity of the brain and is sold as a white odourless powder with a bitter, numbing taste. The powder is extracted from the leaves of the coca bush, found in South America, although street cocaine is usually mixed with impurities like powdered milk, baking powder or bleach.

Cocaine is rapidly absorbed through the mucous membranes lining the nostrils, so it is usually inhaled or snorted through the nose. Sometimes it is injected or smoked.

Its use in Australia has increased in recent years. According to 2010 figures, 7.3 per cent of people have used cocaine at some stage in their lives and 2.1 per cent had used it in the previous 12 months.

SHORT-TERM EFFECTS

Some of the immediate effects include:

- *increased energy and alertness, sometimes agitation*
- *exhilaration*
- *sexual arousal*
- *dilated pupils*
- *loss of appetite*
- *unpredictable behaviour*
- *increased blood pressure and pulse rate*
- *rapid breathing*
- *increased body temperature.*

The 'high' effect from inhaling cocaine lasts for about 30 minutes and is followed by a 'low'.

Using large quantities of cocaine repeatedly within a number of hours can lead to:

- *extreme agitation*
- *hallucinations*
- *unpredictable aggressive behaviour*
- *nausea*
- *vomiting*
- *chest pain*
- *heart attack.*

LONG-TERM EFFECTS

Patients I see who have run into problems with long-term use of cocaine usually present as 'thin, wired and exhausted'. They:

- *have trouble sleeping*
- *become agitated and depressed or paranoid*
- *lose weight*
- *develop nutritional deficiencies.*

Even after a single binge they can have several weeks or months of feeling depressed, lethargic, anxious and 'achey'. They often have an intense craving for cocaine, which can last for several months.

Repeated snorting damages the nasal lining and results in nosebleeds, sinus infections and damage to the tissues between the nostrils.

Using cocaine during pregnancy may cause miscarriage, premature labour or stillbirth.

BENZODIAZEPINES OR 'BENZOS'

I know benzodiazepines are prescription drugs, but there are plenty of people who get into problems with prescribed drugs, and there is also an active black market in the off-label use of benzos. There are more than 30 different prescription drugs in the group, which can often be recognised because their generic name ends in '-azepam', and include Xanax (alprazolam), diazepam (Valium), oxazepam (Serepax), flunitrazepam (Rohypnol) and temazepam (Normison, Nocturne, Euhypnos, Temaze). Medically, they are used to relieve anxiety, relax muscles and induce sleep.

Benzodiazepines slow down the activity of the brain and are highly addictive. The fact that they are provided on prescription from a doctor does not make them any less addictive or potentially dangerous.

In the 2010 National Drug Strategy Household Survey, 1.4 per cent of people had used benzos for non-medical purposes in the past 12 months.

The other pharmaceutical drugs commonly used 'off label' are pain-killers.

SHORT-TERM EFFECTS

Short-term use of benzodiazepines creates an effect of relaxation, calmness, sleepiness and a relief from anxiety. Some people will notice dizziness, blurred or double vision, mood swings, slurred speech, or trouble thinking clearly. If you don't fall asleep, there is an effect similar to being drunk.

Very high doses of benzos can cause unconsciousness or coma, and death in overdose.

LONG-TERM EFFECTS

After just a few weeks or even sooner – sometimes after only a few consecutive days – you can become physically and psychologically dependent on benzos. This is regardless of whether the medication has been medically prescribed or not.

If you use benzos over a long period of time, they can cause a lack of motivation, loss of interest in sex, weight gain, memory loss, irritability, nightmares and trouble sleeping, anxiety and an increased risk of accidents.

Combining benzos with other sedative-type drugs like alcohol, antihistamines, cannabis or heroin increases the sedative effect and can cause unconsciousness, suppress breathing and may be fatal. A number of 'celebrity' deaths have involved benzos in combination with other drugs or alcohol. Even in small doses, it is particularly dangerous if you are driving or operating machinery.

Whether you use benzos medically or recreationally, suddenly stopping the drug after long-term use can cause hallucinations, headaches, confusion, dizziness, insomnia, panic attacks, depression, nausea and vomiting, or seizures. These symptoms eventually subside, but it is much better to reduce the dose gradually over two or three months under medical supervision.

Benzos taken during pregnancy can affect unborn babies and cause them to have to go through a withdrawal after birth.

Hard Drugs

♣ LSD (Lysergic Acid Diethylamide)
People who use one type of drug, such as ecstasy, are likely to use others. In fact, the 2010 National Drug Strategy Household Survey found that 46 per cent of regular ecstasy users had also taken LSD within the past 12 months.

LSD is a powerful hallucinogen, which distorts your perception of reality. It is very unpredictable in dosage and effect.

Effects

- poor coordination
- distorted perception of time, space and self
- vivid hallucinations
- lack of control over thinking
- anxiety
- fear
- depression
- bad trips
- traumatic flashbacks
- impaired memory.

❧ Ice

'Ice' or 'crystal meth' is a crystalline form of methamphetamine. Problems include:

- dependence
- agitation
- weight loss
- disordered thinking
- mental impairment
- depression
- anxiety
- brain damage
- mood swings
- psychosis with paranoia and hallucinations
- heart problems
- malnutrition
- chronic insomnia.

❧ Heroin

Dangers of injecting

If any injection equipment is shared, there is a risk of transmitting HIV, hepatitis B and hepatitis C. Injecting also damages veins.

Effects

- pain relief
- euphoria
- suppression of cough
- sleepiness
- constipation
- nausea
- vomiting
- overdose/death
- risk of HIV and hepatitis B and C if injecting with non-sterile equipment
- impotence in men
- irregular periods and infertility in women.

Heroin users often face family and employment problems and problems with the law.

HARM MINIMISATION

If you are using illicit drugs or legal drugs in a harmful way, you can hurt yourself and others. You may have heard a lot about harm minimisation that, as the name suggests, is about reducing the damage caused by drug-taking. This involves such strategies as needle exchange programs to reduce the transmission of HIV, hepatitis B and hepatitis C in injecting drug users; supervised injecting rooms to reduce overdose deaths; random breath testing to reduce alcohol-related traffic accidents; and naltrexone maintenance and methadone maintenance programs.

Think carefully before you use drugs that will affect your brain. The problems might be immediate and catastrophic, and even occasional use can cause health problems and reduce your potential for ultimate wellness.

There is no way of knowing what ingredients and impurities are in a drug sold in the illicit trade, and there are unexpected accidental overdoses and deaths, even in occasional users. The only sure-fire harm minimisation strategy is to avoid illicit drug use completely.

FOR FURTHER INFORMATION

Contact the NDARC (National Drug and Alcohol Research Centre) http://ndarc.med.unsw.edu.au/

SLEEP

Are you one of those people who, when your head hits the pillow at night you fall fast asleep, sleep soundly for seven or eight hours and wake refreshed and ready to start the day? No? If that doesn't sound like you then we have another clue as to why you might be feeling closer to 50 rather than 100 on the scale of wellness.

It is a well-known fact that sleep deprivation is bad for you, both emotionally and physically. Ask any parent of an unsettled baby or a restless toddler who is up night after night. Interrupted sleep can feel like torture. In fact, sleep deprivation has been used as a form of torture in warfare.

Lack of sleep makes it much harder to cope with day-to-day life. Your body needs sleep to replenish you for each day. If you are not getting enough sleep, sooner or later it shows. Dark circles under the eyes and a pale, drawn face do not paint a picture of good health.

And it is not just a matter of feeling ordinary and looking tired. Chronic lack of sleep has consequences for your health and can even be life-threatening. If you think I am overstating my case, then consider these examples.

The Chernobyl nuclear disaster in 1986 and the *Exxon Valdez* disaster in 1989 were both attributed to overtiredness. But while these major disasters grabbed headlines and shocked us all with the magnitude of the damage they wreaked, chronic sleep deprivation can have both subtle and more obvious impacts on your health and sense of wellbeing.

To be frank, some people don't give themselves a fighting chance at a good night's sleep. They seem to do everything to sabotage their chances, from drinking copious quantities of coffee late into the evening to allowing so little time in bed that they can't hope to get enough hours of quality sleep time, then wonder why they feel exhausted most of the time.

First we will look at the physiology and the nature of normal sleep patterns, then some of the common mistakes people make that lead them to lose sleep. Then we will look at ways of improving your chances of correcting unhealthy sleep patterns.

So, knowing that sleeping is important for your health, how do you get enough of it? From completing the Health Audit (page 15) you will have identified some patterns in your sleep and possibly any issues you can fix to ensure you sleep better. But first you need to work out what might be causing your sleep problems. If you have a restless baby, the answer is simple but there are many other reasons for insomnia.

Understanding the nature of sleep and what can affect it is central to sorting out sleep problems.

STAGES OF SLEEP

Sleep is anything but passive rest for the brain, and the brain has characteristic patterns of activity. There are two main types of sleep: rapid eye movement (REM) sleep and non-REM sleep.

REM sleep was discovered in the 1950s when investigative sleep technology started to be developed. It refers to a stage of sleep where the eyes move rapidly, muscle tone is floppy and heart rate and breathing become irregular. The electroencephalography (EEG), which is the recording of electrical activity along the scalp, shows a rapid low-voltage pattern.

There are four or five episodes of REM sleep each night, with about 90 minutes between the episodes. They last from a few minutes up to 30 or 40 minutes. If you are woken during REM sleep, you may recall vivid dreams.

Non-REM sleep has three stages based on the type of brain activity that occurs during the different stages. Stage 1 is light sleep. You drift in and out of sleep and can easily be roused. You might experience sudden muscle jerks, called 'myoclonic jerks', during this phase. Eyes move slowly and muscle movements slow right down. On the EEG recording, alpha waves disappear and theta waves appear.

During Stage 2 sleep, eye movements stop and brain activity slows. Dreaming rarely occurs during this stage and you can be easily awakened. On the EEG there are some bursts of faster brain waves called 'sleep spindles'.

Stage 3 is characterised by the appearance of very slow brain waves called 'delta waves' mixed with faster waves. These stages represent deep sleep, and it is most difficult to rouse somebody during these stages. There is no eye movement or muscle activity. Dreaming does occur in this stage, although not as much as during REM sleep, and these dreams tend to be less vivid and less memorable. Sleep lightens at the end of each deep sleep phase.

WHAT IS NORMAL SLEEP TIME?

It has been said that Napoleon Bonaparte, Margaret Thatcher and Winston Churchill had something in common: they all got by on just four to six hours' sleep a night. Although I have heard it said that Churchill took daytime naps.

Everyone needs sleep. How much sleep varies a little from person to person and changes with age. Newborn babies sleep at least 18 hours a day. On average, young adults tend to sleep about eight hours. Some people naturally need less sleep – five or six hours – while some show signs of sleep deprivation if they do not get at least eight or nine hours. Elderly people might only sleep an average of six hours a night, but may need a nap during the day.

Virtually all of our body functions operate on rhythms that are governed by the brain and the activity of hormones and other chemical messengers in the body. The main signal for sleep rhythm is exposure of the brain to morning light via the retina and the optic nerve.

The hormone most involved in the rhythm of sleep is melatonin. It is produced by a small gland in the brain called the pineal gland, and secreted from about 9 pm until about 4 am. Maximum sleepiness occurs at around 4 am to 5 am.

For most people, the optimum window for sleep is between 11 pm and 7 am. Going to bed too early or to late may disturb the rhythm.

HOW SLEEP CAN AFFECT YOUR HEALTH

Sleep of sufficient quality and quantity is one of the major contributors to feeling terrific. The corollary to that is lack of sleep can be responsible for a lot of subtle and more overt health problems.

Sometimes there is a 'chicken and egg' situation, where you have to work out whether your ability to achieve wellness is limited because you are not sleeping, or you are not sleeping because you have a health problem that is having an impact on your ability to get quality sleep. Examples of this are obesity causing obstructive sleep apnoea, heart failure causing night-time breathlessness, excessive alcohol consumption, gastro-oesophageal reflux or chronic arthritis pain.

The key to improving sleep quality is often found in addressing these underlying health issues, and then the sleep problem itself can be addressed or will resolve spontaneously.

> ## *Do you have a sleep problem?*
>
> - ❧ It takes you longer than half an hour to get to sleep.
> - ❧ You wake frequently during the night.
> - ❧ You have difficulty staying asleep.
> - ❧ You wake up in the early hours of the morning and have trouble getting back to sleep.
> - ❧ You wake feeling unrefreshed.

SLEEP HYGIENE

Let's start with the fundamentals for a good night's sleep. Experts call this 'sleep hygiene'. We can just call it the good habits for successful sleep.

1. ESTABLISH A COMFORT ZONE

It is amazing how often people complain of sleep problems, yet their sleeping environment is just not conducive to uninterrupted rest. Start with your bedding. Check that you have a comfortable, supportive mattress that is not too old. Make sure the bedclothes are suitable for the weather conditions. If you are too hot or too cold you will not stay comfortable. Bedclothes should be cleaned regularly and the bed made neatly, so it is a pleasant sensory experience to get into bed.

Your pillow needs to be comfortable and able to support your neck.

Next, check the actual room itself. Is it too light or too noisy? If your room seems too light, that can affect your sleep. Arrange to hang dark curtains that block out as much light from the windows as possible. If this is not possible, wearing eye masks may work for you.

If it is noisy, can you move your bed to another part of the house that is quieter, perhaps away from the busy street or noisy neighbours? Earplugs are another possible solution.

Sometimes, and I'm sorry to have to bring this up, the noise is coming from the other person sleeping in the room – a snoring partner. If your lack of sleep is the result of a partner who snores, you have two choices: fix the snoring or move out of the room. It can be a toss-up as to which is worse for the relationship: a tired, sick, over-it grumpy spouse or sleeping solo, especially if you are the snorer and you are blissfully unaware of the torture you are putting everyone else through. It really is a no-brainer though, especially when you consider that successful treatments for snoring are readily available.

The noise in the bedroom can also be coming from a pet. If you share your bedroom with a dog that snorts and snuffles, decides that 3 am is a great time to start self-grooming and barks at every perceived threat, then you might have to make other arrangements for the dog's overnight accommodation.

2. FIX MEDICAL PROBLEMS

Maybe you are restless because you are in pain; for example, from arthritis or back pain. Perhaps you are getting up frequently to go to the toilet. There are many medical reasons for poor sleep, so ask your doctor for help. It is possible that effective treatment is available to relieve your discomfort.

Check all your medications and supplements for side effects that mention insomnia. For example, some people are sensitive to high doses of vitamin B, which will keep them awake. Medications such as steroids, beta-blockers, some antidepressants, appetite suppressants, asthma medications and many others can hype you up or affect sleep quality.

3. EXERCISE

There are masses of reasons why exercise is a good habit to get into, and you can add sleep to the list. Exercise enhances every physiological function: it helps to relieve stress, improve daytime alertness and night-time sleep quality.

The timing is important. Exercising early in the day is best. Afternoons are fine, but get the session finished several hours before your scheduled bedtime. If you exercise later than early evening it can delay the release of the hormone melatonin, which starts the sleep cycle. It also increases your body temperature, and your body needs to cool down in preparation for falling asleep.

Forms of exercise that also incorporate relaxation, such as yoga or tai chi are also beneficial for improving sleep.

4. BEDTIME RITUAL

There are many things that can affect your sleep, including good or bad habits. Falling asleep in front of the television, then finding it hard to get back to sleep once you go to bed, is one of the bad habits.

Set up a bedtime ritual to start the wind-down process. Dim the lights about an hour before you go to bed. Turn off computers, electronic devices, televisions and other sources of light and stimulation. Run a hot bath and add a few drops of lavender oil, then relax and soak in the warmth. Head off to bed when you feel sleepy.

Did your parents repeat the old saying, 'No tears before bedtime', or 'Never let the sun go down on an argument'? It holds true that if you are emotionally upset before you need to go to bed your sleep will be affected, so do not start any difficult conversations where you are likely to have disagreements or arguments. Try to settle any upsets or ill feeling in the household before you go to bed.

Regardless of the time you go to bed, set a regular time for getting up and go outside soon after waking to expose yourself to natural light. Gradually you will find that you feel tired in the evenings at an appropriate time to get enough sleep.

5. NUTRITION

You can get better sleep if you are in a healthy weight range and you restrict kilojoule intake. Limit fatty foods, spicy foods and refined carbohydrates in your diet. Avoid eating large meals too close to bedtime. Include foods rich in tryptophan, such as seaweed products or milk, to boost melatonin levels.

6. ALCOHOL

It is really common to see people 'self-medicating' with alcohol, particularly if they have a few drinks to unwind at the end of the day, or use alcohol as a relaxant. The bad news is that alcohol disrupts your normal sleep patterns and makes snoring and obstructive sleep apnoea worse. So if sleep is a problem for you, then you will need to stay off alcohol or minimise it.

7. CAFFEINE

There can hardly be a person on the planet who doesn't know that caffeine is a stimulant that can keep you awake, but it is important to mention it anyway. Caffeine has long been used inappropriately to keep cramming students up all night studying, or prevent long-distance truck drivers from nodding off on the highway at night. So it is little wonder that drinking caffeine can be a problem for people with sleeping issues. Some people are exquisitely sensitive to caffeine's effect on their ability to sleep.

If you drink a lot of coffee or tea, then you might suffer from withdrawal headaches if you go cold turkey. The best way is to start with cutting out all sources of caffeine – medicinal, coffee, tea, cola drinks, chocolate – after about 3 pm, then work backwards in the day from there, down to an average of zero to two coffees or the equivalent a day, consumed early in the day.

8. NICOTINE

Nicotine is a stimulant that impairs your ability to go into a deep sleep. Smoking also makes snoring worse because it inflames and swells the soft tissues in the nose and throat. If you want a good night's sleep, quit smoking.

9. GET YOUR TIMING RIGHT

Of course if you are not getting to bed until late and you have to get up early the next morning, you are not giving yourself a chance. Set a time limit on watching television or working late so that you have enough time to sleep. You will perform more efficiently the next day.

If you feel tired during the day but you have had lots of sleep, you might be oversleeping. The solution to this is to increase your daily activities and limit sleep to about eight hours at night-time.

10. RESOLVE WORRIES OF THE DAY

If you go to sleep at night with unresolved issues on your mind, you could be worrying yourself awake. Problems always loom larger at night, so you need to find a way to block worrying thoughts. Try to put your concerns into perspective. If there is a problem at work and you have yourself convinced that it will end your career, then you need to take a reality check. Take a mental step back and think, 'How real is my concern?', 'What is the *likely* outcome?' Then replace your negative 'doom and gloom' thoughts with a positive one.

If something is weighing on your mind, try to discuss it with a family member, friend or work colleague early in the evening and then put it on the 'to do' list for tomorrow. Consider whether you can constructively do something about this concern right now, or even before morning. If not, write yourself a note and put the thought aside until the next day.

If you are wide awake, try putting a mental shield between you and your worries. Then imagine yourself in the place you have felt the most relaxed. Maybe it is on a beach, or a ski slope, or somewhere you once had a relaxing holiday.

Stressful life events such as job loss, financial problems or relationship difficulties can increase your body's production of stress hormones such as cortisol and adrenaline. Anxiety and depression can also show up as sleep problems. Conversely, sleep problems can create or exacerbate depression. Counselling may help you to resolve these issues.

❧ PSYCHOLOGICAL THERAPIES

Cognitive behavioural therapy (CBT) is a psychological technique that helps you to change established thinking and behaviour patterns, particularly if you have developed negative ideas about trying to sleep that cause you anxiety. CBT is very effective in treating chronic insomnia, and is usually taught by a psychologist trained in the technique.

Counselling can also help to work through practical solutions to problems that are causing you to feel anxious. If you have had a death in the family, you are going through a divorce, you have problems with your children or your marriage, or financial worries, talking to friends, family members, your GP, a psychologist or a counsellor will help.

❧ RELAXATION

Establish a relaxed and stress-free mood in the house. Put on some quiet, cruisy music. Avoid arguments or tension or sources of stress. Finish up any work at least an hour before you go to bed, which means turning off the computer. Make an effort to learn some relaxation techniques such as stretching, meditation, breathing techniques or visualisation. Regular massage has a relaxing effect, which can also help to relieve muscle tension.

11. SEE THE LIGHT!

Well-timed light stimulation can help reset your body rhythms. For example, trouble getting to sleep may be helped by exposure to bright morning light. In climates where it does not get light until later in the morning, you may need to use an artificial bright light source.

People who get sleepy early in the evening but wake up very early in the morning may benefit from exposure to light in the early evening along with some gentle exercise.

❧ ACUPUNCTURE

Acupuncture works for a lot of people who have insomnia. The evidence is not overwhelming, but individuals do report success with it. It might be worth trying.

❧ MELATONIN

Melatonin is the hormone secreted at night by the pineal gland near the brain, which gives the signal to sleep. It is sometimes used for a few weeks to reset the sleep rhythm, and is probably more effective as a therapy in older people. It is commonly used by international travellers to combat jet lag and by shift workers needing to reset their body clocks.

It is a good idea to ask for medical advice about the timing and dosage of melatonin. For example, if you have trouble getting to sleep, a dose of 0.3–5 mg of melatonin can be taken in the early evening to help you fall to sleep earlier.

If waking in the early hours of the morning is your problem, early evening exposure to light and melatonin taken when you wake around 3–5 am will help you to sleep longer in the morning.

Tryptophan is a precursor to melatonin, so tryptophan-rich foods such as seaweed products or warm milk can boost melatonin levels.

Checklist for a great night's sleep

- ❧ Reduce noise.
- ❧ Darken the room.
- ❧ Check you have a comfortable, supportive mattress that is not too old.
- ❧ Make sure you have a comfortable pillow that supports your neck.
- ❧ Exercise early in the day, finishing at least a few hours before bedtime.
- ❧ Arrange medical treatment for conditions that might affect sleep, such as chronic pain management.
- ❧ Ask your doctor or pharmacist to check all of your medications for the possibility they could affect sleep.
- ❧ Avoid drinking excessive alcohol as it affects sleep quality.
- ❧ Do not drink or eat anything containing caffeine after midafternoon.
- ❧ Do not smoke. Nicotine is a stimulant and affects sleep quality, so this includes all forms of nicotine replacement.
- ❧ Avoid taking pharmaceutical sedatives or other medications except in the very short term.
- ❧ Plan your next day and talk through any problems or issues long before you go to bed, and try not to go to bed angry or upset.
- ❧ Dim the lights in the house an hour before bedtime.
- ❧ Have a bedtime ritual. Perhaps try a hot bath, a drink of hot milk, put on some quiet music and do some relaxation exercises.
- ❧ Give yourself enough hours in bed to get the sleep you need.
- ❧ Don't be too rigid about your bedtime, but avoid going to bed way too early or very late.
- ❧ Do not sleep with pets in the room if they disturb you.
- ❧ Set the alarm so you get up at a regular time.
- ❧ Avoid daytime naps of longer than 20 minutes.

❧ HERBAL THERAPIES

Common herbal treatments for insomnia include the following:

- **Valerian** *is very popular as an insomnia treatment; it is usually used in combination with other herbs, such as hops, lavender, skullcap,* *passionflower and lemon balm. It may reduce the time it takes to get to sleep and improve sleep quality. You need to be patient though, as the effect may not kick in for about two weeks.*

- **Lavender** *has a relaxing effect and can reduce anxiety and improve mood, concentration and sleep.*
- **Lemon balm** *is often prescribed in combination with other herbs such as valerian.*
- **Chamomile tea** *would be worth trying to see if it helps you. There is not much evidence for chamomile tea in insomnia treatment but it does seem to have a mild sedative effect and is safe.*

Some sleep disorders will need to be referred to a specialist sleep clinic for advanced treatment techniques. Whatever the cause of your insomnia, there are ways of dealing with it, so there is no need to put up with the torture of sleep deprivation.

INSOMNIA

Insomnia can exhibit itself in a variety of ways. You might have trouble getting to sleep, staying asleep or getting enough quality sleep. It may be a result of bad habits, life stresses or a symptom of anxiety or depression.

MANAGING INSOMNIA

✿ MEDICATION

A warning about medication for insomnia: medications such as benzo-diazepines – Normison (temazepam), Valium (diazepam), Rohypnol (flunitrazepam), and Mogadon – and related medications have their place in the very short term but addiction is common and over time you find you need higher doses to have the same effect, so they should be avoided for more long-term treatment.

The drug Zolpidem has some emerging reports of serious and bizarre side effects and I would advise you to avoid it.

A lot of patients try to negotiate with their doctors for inappropriate prescription of medications for insomnia. The overuse or the inappropriate use of sedatives is common. Such is the distress that is caused by lack of sleep, it is easy to understand the desperation that stems from trying to 'just fix it'.

Taking a sedative for a few days here and there can be part of a short-term solution to a short-term problem, but it is not the comprehensive solution you need. Very few people who use 'sleeping pills' regularly will experience an improvement in their sleep problem in the long term and, in fact, many find that their sleeping problem gets worse with time. Sooner or later, tolerance to the drugs can develop so that increased doses or stronger drugs are needed to get the same effect.

There have been multiple media reports of one sleeping pill, Zolpidem, causing bizarre night-time behaviours that the person is completely unable to recall. Such is the dependence on these sorts of medications that even these known adverse side effects do not deter people from seeking a prescription for them.

Sleep disorders are associated with:

* daytime fatigue
* impaired memory
* impaired alertness
* poor coordination
* irritability and depressed mood
* high blood pressure
* obesity
* diabetes
* increased risk of stroke
* heart, immune system and endocrine dysfunction
* increased number of accidents.

Also worrying is that the inappropriate use of sedatives such as the benzodiazepines commonly leads to dependence, depression, mental dullness and worsening of fatigue. Taking them can be particularly dangerous for elderly people, who are more likely to have a fall if they have to get up at night to go to the bathroom while they are under the influence of medication. Sedatives can also exaggerate any decline in cognitive ability.

Masking the symptom of insomnia with sedatives also does nothing to address the underlying cause. The most effective treatment will depend to a large extent on the type and cause of your sleep disorder. The right treatment program may take more effort than swallowing a pill, but the effort is worth the long-term result.

Where a sleep disorder is your fundamental problem, regardless of the type of sleep disorder, the signs and symptoms of sleep deprivation have a big impact on your health-related quality of life.

SLEEP DISORDERS NEEDING MEDICAL ATTENTION

Some sleep problems happen because of a physical or psychological problem and amount to a version of simple insomnia. Other times it is the culmination of bad habits, which can be reversed with simple lifestyle changes and some effort to address the problem.

More serious sleep disorders call for medical diagnosis and intervention. There are some symptoms and signs of more serious sleep disorders that signal that you should talk to your doctor.

Warnings signs of a possible sleep disorder needing medical attention

- stopping breathing during sleep, with gasping, choking sounds or heavy snoring
- daytime fatigue and nodding off
- sudden attacks of sleep
- kicking about in sleep
- aching, jumpy restless feeling in legs at night
- sleepwalking
- night terrors with screaming and apparent terror
- teeth grinding

OBSTRUCTIVE SLEEP APNOEA (OSA)

Who in the old days would have thought snoring could be a health risk, beyond the effect of a solid thump from your sleep-deprived partner? We now know that if you snore loudly, and particularly in a pattern of stop–start breathing characteristic of a condition called obstructive sleep apnoea (OSA), you should have it investigated and treated as a priority issue. Some people with sleep apnoea can stop breathing hundreds of times a night for up to a minute, causing not only disturbed quality of sleep but also strain on your heart and reduced oxygen to the brain.

We also know that the stereotypical snorer – male, middle-aged, overweight, smoker, heavy drinker – is far from the only image of a problem snorer. And although it is far more common in men than women, snoring problems and OSA can affect either gender. Virtually any age, male or female, and any body shape can be affected.

In childhood the most common cause of snoring and OSA is enlarged tonsils and/or adenoids. If your snoring child is tired or irritable during the day, or their school performance is declining, don't put it down to laziness or naughtiness – they need to be assessed with a sleep study.

Adults can also have blocked upper airways such as sinus problems or blocked nasal passages due to polyps or hay fever. The most common problem area is the soft palate at the back of the throat, which vibrates loudly as air passes in when inhaling.

Obesity is probably the most significant issue, especially in people who are carrying weight around the neck. You gain fat on the inside as well as the outside, and that increased thickness of tissue in the throat and the back of the nose decreases the opening of the airways.

Snoring is definitely worse in smokers because of swelling due to inflammation of the nasal passages and throat tissues, and heavy drinkers because of excessive relaxation of the muscles of the airways.

The implications can be serious. Not only does disturbed sleep result in daytime sleepiness and lethargy, it can start to affect your mood and personality, your ability to concentrate, increase the rate of accidents, reduce libido and cause morning headaches and high blood pressure.

You need a formal sleep study to confirm OSA and distinguish it from other causes of snoring or daytime sleepiness. The next step is to treat the causes and contributory factors. This might mean a serious and sustained attempt at weight loss, nasal or sinus surgery, reducing alcohol intake, or quitting smoking. Some people swear by anti-snoring pillows or mouthguard-type dental devices. You could try those.

More severe cases of OSA will need to consider the immediate use of a device called a continuous positive airway pressure pump or CPAP, a type of breathing apparatus that fits over your face and is strapped to your head, attached by tubing to a pump device that forces airflow into the mouth and nose, keeping the airways of the throat and pharynx open. Not the thing for spontaneous fits of passion in the wee small hours but it might just save your life – and your relationship.

NARCOLEPSY

Narcolepsy is a rare neurological disorder that typically starts in adolescence or young adulthood. People with narcolepsy are overcome by an overwhelming sense of falling asleep in the daytime, which might be accompanied by sudden loss of muscle tone and even collapse.

Narcolepsy usually needs to be treated with medications and lifestyle changes, and avoiding caffeine and alcohol within six hours of bedtime.

MOVEMENT DISORDERS

🍃 RESTLESS LEGS SYNDROME

This is a condition where your legs feel jumpy and restless at night and you just can't keep them still. It is more common in women than in men. There may be an underlying medical problem.

This syndrome can be treated with exercise early in the day, hot baths, magnesium supplements and correcting any iron deficiency. Sometimes medication is needed.

🍃 PERIODIC LIMB MOVEMENTS

These are short bursts of sudden movement of the legs and sometimes the arms during sleep. Usually you are unaware of the movements unless they wake you, but a sleeping partner will report it and may be disturbed by it.

Once the diagnosis is established, treatment involves removing all stimulants such as nicotine and caffeine, and managing any sources of stress.

🍃 TEETH GRINDING AND CLENCHING

This often shows up to dentists and doctors as headaches, jaw pain or worn-down teeth. It can disturb the deeper stages of sleep and is most common in childhood.

Treatment involves removing stimulants – caffeine, alcohol, drugs – and managing stress. Teeth may need to be protected with a splint worn between the upper and lower jaw at night.

❧ SLEEP TERRORS AND SLEEPWALKING

Sleep terrors and sleepwalking usually happen between one and three hours after going to sleep, and occur during non-REM sleep stages. They are the result of partial arousal from slow-wave sleep. The events usually cannot be remembered. They are both associated with lack of sleep, erratic sleep schedules and life stresses.

Treatment involves stress management, establishing a regular sleep pattern and addressing general sleep routines.

❧ NIGHTMARES

Nightmares usually happen during REM sleep. Treatment involves reducing life stresses, getting treatment for anxiety, avoiding excess alcohol, and avoiding the use of night sedatives.

MOVING FORWARD

Here are a few ideas from me for goals to set yourself regarding sleep.

GOALS

- *To fall asleep without difficulty.*
- *To sleep undisturbed or with just one or two waking times in the night, but getting back to sleep without difficulty.*
- *To wake refreshed, feeling as though I have had enough quality sleep.*

YOUR GOALS

Goal	Activity	Obstacles/solutions	Result
To get better quality sleep	Create a more comfortable bedroom. Get up at the same time every day	Get overstressed about not sleeping well: make sleep more of a priority	Sleeping undisturbed

NUTRITION

I suspect I know what you're thinking: 'I can just skim this chapter or skip it altogether because I know everything there is to know about diets. You name a diet, I've been on it and none of them works for more than a few weeks.'

Or maybe you are thinking, 'I eat well. I'm not overweight or underweight. I don't need to know any more about nutrition.'

Well, you may need to think again.

There is a vast chasm of difference between knowing what you ought to be eating and what you actually do eat. You may have a 'perfect' diet, consistent and finely balanced, have stacks of energy, adjust your food intake to match your activity level and your weight sits within the healthy weight range. If so, well done. If not, then you have a facet of your life that is within your power to improve, if you are to reach your goal of ultimate wellness.

It is also likely that since you are reading a book about how to achieve ultimate wellness, you recognise you are not feeling all that great but you know that you just might be able to improve your health and wellbeing by making some realistic changes.

I am not going to talk to you about 'dieting' per se. What I have to say has to do with the quantity of food and nutrients you put into your body, and also the quality of nutrition. I also want to say a few things about how the way you think about food ultimately affects and is affected by how you feel about yourself.

Being in a healthy weight range is important for your overall wellbeing and a good indicator for how healthy you are, so in view of the global epidemic of obesity, I will discuss weight loss in this chapter. But the focus here is nutrition and how the food you eat affects your health. I want to talk to you about how food affects how you feel on the inside, not just how you look on the outside.

ASSESSING YOUR DIET AND WEIGHT AS INDICATORS OF YOUR HEALTH

INTERPRETING YOUR BMI AND WAIST MEASUREMENTS

In the Health Audit (page 15), you will have measured and recorded your height, weight, body mass index (BMI) and waist circumference. Looking at these results will give you some idea of how healthy your weight is in a medical sense. If your measurements have led you to conclude you are underweight or overweight, you can consider what sort of action you might want to take.

BEING OVERWEIGHT/OBESE

There is an epidemic of obesity in many countries in the world. The World Health Organization estimates that 65 per cent of the world's population live in countries where being overweight or obese kills more people than being underweight and overall, more than one in ten of the world's adult population is obese. Being overweight or obese is associated with an increased risk of dozens of chronic diseases.

If you are overweight or obese, you have a greater chance of developing high blood pressure, high blood cholesterol, type 2 diabetes, heart disease, stroke, osteoarthritis and certain cancers. So, making the decision to take off weight is a crucial element in your plan to achieve ultimate wellness.

There is a direct link between waist measurement and increased risk of several types of cancer, in particular cancer of the colon, prostate, postmenopausal breast cancer, and cancers of the endometrium, kidney and oesophagus. Although it seems inconsistent, many people who are overweight are also suffering from malnutrition and nutritional deficiencies.

If you are a man with a waist measurement over 100 cm or a woman with a waist measurement over 85 cm, then your risk for cancer is increased.

Waist measurement has also been linked with other health risks, such as type 2 diabetes and cardiovascular disease. An elevated waist–hip ratio is a strong predictor of heart attack, even after other risk factors are taken into account.

Upon taking these measurements, you may want to lose some weight and adjust your diet to improve your health. The information in this chapter will help you to reassess your eating habits and refine your diet to be more nutritionally balanced.

BEING UNDERWEIGHT

Because of the epidemic of being overweight and obesity, the problem of being underweight is often overlooked. There are significant health problems associated with being under the healthy weight range. Eating disorders such as anorexia nervosa are well recognised. Where a significant eating disorder is causing you to be underweight, intensive and specialised treatment is required. Some people just have trouble putting weight on or keeping it on. Being underweight increases your risk of poor immune function, respiratory disease, gut disease, dry skin and hair, hair loss, fatigue, irritability, weakness and osteoporosis. It is also associated with an increased risk of falls and fractures. Being underweight means you are more likely to be deficient in protein and essential vitamins and minerals as well.

This chapter will help you assess your eating behavior and food attitudes to increase body weight to your healthy range. If you are having trouble gaining weight because of a medical problem, or because you are not able to gain weight despite increasing your food intake, I would advise you to keep a food diary and photograph a typical plate; then see a dietitian to analyse your food quantities and nutritional content of your diet.

QUALITY OF YOUR DIET

In my clinical practice as a doctor, I always ask patients about their diets. This is because it is not possible to gain a full insight into a patient's health without assessing the fuel that is going into the tank. As you would expect, I get a huge range of responses. A common conversation goes like this:

Patient: 'We eat really well. The wife cooks most nights. You know, meat or chicken and a few veggies.'

Patient's partner: 'You might eat well when you are at home, but you're not counting the business lunches and all the chocolate you have after dinner.'

Patient: 'I don't eat that much chocolate. Doctor, how much chocolate is okay?'

Me: 'A couple of squares of dark chocolate a day would be okay.'

[Pause.]

Patient's partner: 'So you would not consider a half a family block of milk chocolate every night to be "healthy"?'

Me: 'We may have just found our first clue to why your cholesterol is a bit high.'

Another scenario might go like this:

Patient: 'I am exhausted all the time. I get the kids off to school and I could just go back to bed for a couple of hours.'

Me: 'Tell me about your diet.'

Patient: 'Well, there's no problem there! I know a lot about diets. I have been on so many of them. For the last few months I have been on that great Paleolithic diet. You know, the natural caveman one.'

Me: 'So you are eating a lot of fruit and nuts?'

Patient: 'No. I sort of modified it from the Dukan diet, that one that's only meat in the beginning.'

Me: 'So you are eating just meat and no grains?'

Patient: 'And a little bit of fruit.'

Me: 'Any problem with constipation or bad breath?'

Patient: 'I take something for the bowels, but my breath is okay.'

Patient's partner: 'Um. I haven't said anything but it's not that flash. And you are cranky *all* the time.'

Or this:

Patient's mother: 'She wants to sleep all day. She can't concentrate at school. She is constantly complaining about being tired no matter how much sleep she gets.'

Me (to patient): 'Tell me about your diet.'

Patient: 'I'm a vegetarian.'

Me: 'Who else is vegetarian in your family?'

Patient's mother: 'Just her. It's a phase. She visited a friend's farm in the holidays and ever since she has refused to eat anything that once had a pulse. She refuses to eat eggs too because they were going to be chickens.'

Me: 'So you do the food preparation? What do you make her?'

Patient's mother: 'She just has whatever we're having but without the meat or chicken or fish.'

Me: 'Do you make tofu?'

Patient's mother: 'Wouldn't have a clue what to do with it.'

Me (to patient): 'When did you start your periods?'

Patient: 'When I was 13.'

Me: 'What foods do you eat that have iron or protein in them?'

Patient: [Blank look, shrugs shoulders.] 'Dunno.'

THE FOOD DIARY

One of the first things I ask patients to do for a nutritional assessment is a detailed audit of their actual diet, as you have done with the food diary in the Health Audit (page 15). If you are like most people, when your doctor or dietitian asks you about your diet you most likely tell them about an idealised diet, what you know you should be saying, or what you might eat on a 'perfect' day, leaving out the odd snacks and junk food and grazing.

So the best thing about doing the food diary accurately is that it will show you the diet you are actually eating and not just the one you would prefer to tell your doctor about. It's an almost sure bet that it won't be the diet you know you should be eating to stay healthy. But from this honest record keeping, you can properly evaluate your diet.

Accurately documenting a few days of eating and drinking gives you the information you need to analyse what you are actually eating and drinking, and then you can work out a practical plan for how you could improve the content of your diet, and overcome any obstacles you might face. By assessing what you are eating and what you are not eating, you may realise you are manifestly deficient in a key nutritional area, like carbohydrates or protein or iron. Or perhaps you will see a pattern of skipping meals and snacking later in the day.

Case study

David is a businessman who was finding it hard to lose weight. We talked about his diet, and certainly on the surface it seemed as though there wasn't a lot of room for improvement. I asked him to keep a food diary and to see me again in a week. After three days he called me and said, 'I discovered the problem on day one. I have a wonderful secretary who fusses around after me. She makes me about six cups of tea a day, no sugar of course. Keeping the food diary, I noticed that with every cup of tea she brought me two biscuits, which I just ate at my desk.' We figured out that 12 biscuits a day, five days a week added up to 60 biscuits. All David had to do was cut out 50 of them and the weight he wanted to lose came off easily.

Once you have completed your food diary, take a good hard look at what it reveals:

- *What patterns can you see?*
- *Do you tend to miss any meals?*
- *How many pieces of fruit do you eat every day?*
- *How many serves of vegetables every day?*
- *What are your sources of protein?*
- *Do you snack? What do you use for snacks, and what quantities?*
- *What processed or packaged foods do you eat?*
- *How much alcohol do you drink?*
- *How much water do you drink?*

MINDFUL EATING

One value of keeping a food diary is the information you gather in recording what you actually eat and drink, and the other advantage is that it encourages 'mindful eating'. When I am reinforcing the value of a food diary, I will point out to patients that it is as therapeutic as it is informative. And here's why. In writing down everything you eat and drink, you become really aware of your eating behaviours. You become, literally, mindful of what you are doing. Once you know the principles of healthy eating, then the food diary reminds you constantly to think about whether a particular choice is healthy for you because you know the aim of the exercise is to record it all.

Put simply, mindfulness is deliberately paying attention, non-judgementally, to what is going on in your internal and external environment. It is a technique used to help you overcome all sorts of automatic, habitual patterns of thinking, feeling and acting.

Learning 'mindful eating' involves a number of elements:

- *deliberately paying attention to the positive elements of the experience of food preparation and eating*
- *choosing to eat food that you enjoy and that is nourishing to your body*
- *using all your senses to explore, savour and taste*
- *simply noting your responses to food – like/take-it-or-leave-it/dislike*
- *becoming aware of your mind and body cues that you are hungry and need to eat*

- *becoming aware of your mind and body cues that you have eaten enough and it is time to stop eating.*

With time, the aim of mindful eating is to develop an awareness of your immediate responses to food, then gain insight into how your momentary food choices affect how you feel while you are preparing and eating food, and ultimately, an awareness of your food choices on your specific longer term health goals.

MINDLESS EATING

Recording everything you eat forces you to think about what you are doing at the time. In one respect, its opposite could be called 'mindless eating', where you just graze or nibble on food because it's there. I see a lot of mothers of young children who do this while they are preparing their children's afternoon tea and dinner. They graze on whatever they are preparing, then prepare and eat another meal when their partner gets home.

Sometimes mindless eating is a result of being bored or distracted, like the bowl of nuts or the bar of chocolate you nibble through while you watch the television. It is easy to get into the habit of eating mindlessly if you are working at a computer and you have snacks on the desk. You will be concentrating on the work you are doing and automatically pick up small amounts of food, which all stacks up the kilojoules.

REBOOT YOUR ATTITUDE TO FOOD

There has long been a fascination for fad diets promising almost instantaneous results, usually for weight loss. Entire industries have been built around fad diet concepts. Over the years we have heard about the Israeli Army diet, the Atkins diet, the South Beach diet, the Pritikin diet, the Blood Type diet, the Paleolithic diet and many more. I get asked about them all the time.

The reasons I have a problem with most fad diets is that they encourage an unhealthy obsession with one element of nutrition, usually weight loss, and many of the fad diets promoted by celebrities or the media are not nutritionally balanced or sustainable in the long term.

One of the common reactions I get when I suggest that we look at dietary changes to achieve a health goal is, 'I hate diets. I have been on every diet ever invented and nothing works. I don't want to go on another diet.'

We need to redefine 'dieting'. The word has come to be synonymous with 'cruel and unusual punishment', especially for people who are 'foodies'. A restrictive fad diet that cuts out all or most of the foods you love is not the intention.

So how about we turn the concept of fad dieting into a positive; something you can look forward to as a catalyst for change. Dieting, if you do it at all, needs to be a short-term exercise with a finite aim. The positive focus of short-term dieting is to reboot your attitude to food.

Rather than tut-tutting about fad diets, which as a doctor you would expect to be my usual default position, I recognise they can fulfil a constructive, if short-term, objective. Fad diets get you to focus your thinking on food, something you probably do not do often unless you have a specific problem such as a food allergy. They also force you to get out of a rut, change your established eating patterns, even if only for few weeks. It is not so much the weeks or months you are on a fad diet that will have the lasting effect.

Look at it this way: a fad diet is really a crash course in mindful eating. The genuine challenge is to transition the fad, or the novel eating pattern, into a long-term nutrition solution. In other words, eating the right combination, quality and balance of food needs to become your usual pattern. Your new normal.

NEW FAD DIET ALERT!!
Eat Breakfast and Pack Your Own Lunch Diet!

EATING PATTERNS

One of the big problems I see with eating patterns is the number of people who skip breakfast and then eat whatever they can get their hands on for lunch. That means you are a captive of whatever takeaway food is available around your workplace.

Actually, I think I might start a fad diet of my own.

I will call it the 'Eat Breakfast and Pack Your Own Lunch Diet'. If you just did that, ate breakfast every day and packed lunch on workdays so that even on your busiest days you had those meals covered, then a large proportion of diet-related problems like lack of energy, trouble losing weight, being underweight or snacking on all the wrong foods would be solved.

BREAKFAST

My first question for you is this: Do you eat breakfast? Notice I didn't ask *what* you have for breakfast. What you have for breakfast is my second question, which presumes you do eat *something* for breakfast.

Many people don't eat breakfast regularly. Even working mothers who make breakfast and pack lunches for their children skip this essential part of their daily routine in their morning rush.

Why am I harping on about breakfast? There is an old saying that breakfast is the most important meal of the day. I know this is going to sound really obvious, but you need food for energy. Not just for the going to the gym, running-a-marathon type energy, but the type of energy where you feel like bouncing out of bed in the morning, your brain is firing, and you feel motivated and animated and ready for all the challenges the day brings.

Attention, concentration, memory and work performance are optimised if you eat in the morning. And if you are inclined to unstable moods at all, then eating breakfast will contribute to a steadier mood state.

Reasons to eat breakfast regularly

Breakfast:
- restores your blood sugar levels from the overnight fast
- restores vitamin and mineral levels
- improves concentration and work performance
- gives you more energy
- helps control your body weight
- stabilises mood
- combats fatigue
- encourages other healthy behaviours
- reduces unhealthy snacking later in the day.

If you want to keep your weight in the healthy range, then this is another reason to eat breakfast. At any age, if you skip breakfast you are more likely to eat more later in the day and to be overweight.

A Taiwanese study found that adolescents who ate breakfast regularly were less likely to be overweight, and that the odds of becoming overweight were 51 per cent greater for those who ate breakfast irregularly. Irregular breakfast eaters were also less likely to have other healthy behaviours.

If you do skip breakfast, you probably have one of the common excuses for doing so: there is not enough time, there is nothing to eat in the house, or you are too tired or rushed to bother. I've heard them all. But they each have a simple solution.

'I don't have time in the morning,' is the most common reason. If this is you, try this exercise. Set your alarm just 10 or 15 minutes earlier and get up. Use a stopwatch to time how long it takes, from start to finish, to put cereal and milk in a bowl and grab a piece of fruit and eat it. Of course, it takes no more than a few minutes. You can save even more time by putting a bowl and spoon out on the kitchen bench the night before.

Like most things in life, creating a breakfast routine takes a little preparation. You can't make toast if you don't have bread in the house. You can't have cereal if there is none in the pantry or you forgot to pick up the milk. So remember to set up a routine of shopping for the next day so that simple breakfast foods are in the house each morning.

'But I'm so rushed. I prefer to grab breakfast on the way to work,' is another one I hear. This story plays itself out all the time. One common scenario is the busy executive who grabs a jumbo coffee and two pieces of buttered raisin toast or a slab of banana bread on the way to work, bursts in the door of the office and wolfs everything down while the computer is booting up. While something is better than nothing, this 'fast food' breakfast is high in kilojoules, saturated fat and refined sugar. More fat if there is full-fat milk in the coffee.

Or the other one: 'I can't be bothered eating before I get to work.' Maybe you are one of those people who plans to prepare breakfast when you get to the office. You might think it is more convenient but there are a number of pitfalls with this plan:

- *You get to work and the phone is ringing and you have to hit the ground running. The next moment you have time to eat is after 11.*
- *You may run out of cereal or milk, someone may accidentally eat your food and not all offices appreciate their staff preparing food during office hours.*

- *Worst of all, eating at your desk while you are doing something else tends to be 'mindless eating'.*

Eating at work or on the way to work is not the best way to engage in mindful eating at breakfast. The only sure way of getting a good, nutritious breakfast is to eat before you leave home.

Foods to keep in the house for breakfast

- ❧ cereal
- ❧ milk
- ❧ fruit

- ❧ yoghurt
- ❧ bread
- ❧ eggs

Most of these items last a week in the refrigerator or pantry, so a weekly shopping trip would take care of these basic supplies.

LUNCH

Many of my patients describe lunch as 'whatever I can pick up as takeaway near the office'. This means that lunch varies enormously depending on what is available within easy walking distance of your workplace. One of the obstacles to healthy lunches is not being able to find healthy takeaway alternatives in the close vicinity of your office or workplace. Another common pattern is to skip lunch altogether, with the possible exception of a coffee or three, and grab something to eat on the run at about 3 pm or 4 pm.

A simple solution to this problem is the most obvious one. Pack your own lunch.

Like breakfast, packing your own lunch requires a little planning in food shopping, but something as simple as a bread roll, a small tin of tuna and some chopped salad veggies, and grabbing a piece of fruit is all you need. Lunch for one on the run. Another easy option is to make a little extra food the night before and take the leftovers with you for lunch the next day.

Other patients I see are business people who use the 'business lunch' as a way of meeting and schmoozing clients. The business lunch is also used as an excuse for a three-course meal with wine in the middle of a working day.

This is a time for 'mindful ordering'. When you are ordering food in the middle of the day, think about your activity level for that day and what you are planning to eat for dinner. Try to order food based on what you have decided is right for you, according to your healthy eating principles, and not on what the people with you are eating and drinking. Think about whether or not you want to drink alcohol during your working day. If not, you could simply decline and ask for water, or make the excuse, 'I don't drink in the middle of the day.'

DINNER

It might be easy to grab takeaway, but a lot of takeaway contains hidden ingredients, like unhealthy fats, salt and sugar, which you would, hopefully, not put into your home-cooked food. However, just cooking at home doesn't guarantee nutritional quality either.

So what are some of the solutions to have you preparing more healthy meals at home?

- *One of the best things about the explosion in television cooking shows is that they teach a skill that was at risk of being lost: home cooking. Find a cooking show that interests you and record it so you can play back the vision. Download the recipes from the internet, watch the cooking techniques and try it yourself. I find it very useful to have just a few carefully selected recipe books, websites or apps with quick and easy recipes to give me ideas on broadening my cooking repertoire.*

- *If you really have no idea how to cook, then look for a cooking class or ask a friend or family member who knows how to cook to show you some basics.*

- *Many people cite 'lack of time' as their main reason for not cooking at home. Like the earlier meals in the day, dinner also takes planning and you need to make it a priority and find the time. It's really just as simple as having the raw ingredients in your refrigerator and pantry, thinking ahead about what you are going to cook and doing the shopping either ahead of time or regularly during the week in preparation. You don't need to be an aspiring Michelin star chef to cook at home, but you do need to be organised.*

- *On a practical level, make sure you have the right basic equipment,*

including a stove and oven that work, pots and pans and utensils, and a
pantry stocked with basic supplies.

- *When you are thinking about what to include in a balanced meal plan, think about a source of protein (lean meat, chicken, fish, eggs, legumes, tofu) and carbohydrate, a wide variety of vegetables, herbs and spices. Think fibre and remember to include omega-3 fatty acids.*

- *If you are inclined to eat out at night, remember not to eat too heavy a meal. Many restaurants these days have healthy low-fat options or will modify dishes to accommodate special requests. Avoiding the bread roll, ordering sauces on the side rather than on your meal and sharing a dessert are old tricks of the trade.*

MINDFUL SNACKING

A 'snack' is a small portion of food you eat at times other than your regular established mealtimes. A snack will prevent you becoming over-hungry between meals and helps you to manage your appetite at mealtimes. Like your other meals, snacking needs to be planned and mindful.

The right type and timing of snacks are important. Even if you look after your diet at breakfast, lunch and dinner, snacks can be your weak link.

There are smart choices and not-so-smart choices for snacks. Smart choices are small portions of fruit, low-fat yoghurt, nuts, hummus or vegetable dips with rice crackers, or fresh, chopped vegetables. Not-so-smart choices are the ones with high kilojoule content or energy density but low nutrient quality, like packets of chips, lollies, packaged biscuits, or donuts. Water is a much smarter choice than soft drink or fruit juice.

I want to take this opportunity to warn you off diet drinks as a way of losing weight. Research suggests that drinking diet soda is actually associated with a greater rate of weight gain and increased waist circumference. In addition, the artificial sweeteners often used in diet products (such as aspartame) can cause adverse reactions in some people.

NUTRITIONAL BASICS

As you assess and consider what changes you might like to make to your diet to either help you lose weight and/or improve your health, you need to look beyond the kilojoule content and consider closely whether your diet covers the nutritional basics. I have noticed that patients are increasingly asking me more detailed questions about the effect of nutrition on their health and disease management, which foods to include or avoid, and whether supplements would be useful for them.

There is a growing awareness of the role of micronutrients, food safety and food quality in health. Before we get into the finer details, we need to cover the basics of nutrition, because that is where I see most of the problems occurring, and most of the benefits to be gained.

❧ DIET COMPONENTS

Referring to your food diary, look at the timing of your meals and snacks, then look at their nutritional quality. If you check any guide to balanced nutrition, you will find the same basic list of foods to include.

Fruit

Fewer than half of Australians eat the recommended two pieces of fruit a day. Regularly eating fruit reduces your risk of heart disease, type 2 diabetes, some cancers and macular degeneration. Fruit would have to be the easiest and fastest 'fast food' there is. You can grab it and run, or slice up a banana to put on your breakfast cereal. That's why it is hard to understand why fewer than half of Australians eat the recommended two pieces of fruit a day. To get the greatest benefit, try to eat whole fruit because fresh fruit contains more fibre and fewer concentrated kilojoules than fruit juice.

Vegetables and legumes

The current health recommendation is for five serves of vegetables a day and, like with fruit, most people struggle to eat their quota every day. Raw or cooked vegetables can be used as snack food or as part of lunch and dinner. Salad vegetables can be used as a sandwich filling. Vegetable soup can make a healthy lunch. Stir-fries, vegetable patties and vegetable curries make nutritious evening meals. Try cutting up raw vegetables like carrot and celery sticks, or cucumber with hummus for a snack 'on the run'.

Lean meat, fish, poultry, eggs, nuts, legumes and tofu

These can all provide protein. It is easy to incorporate a source of protein into snacks and meals. You need to get the right proportion of protein in your diet, not too little or too much. Diets that are too low in protein will leave you lacking in energy, emotionally unstable and having trouble concentrating. Your immune system might suffer. You may suffer hair loss, weak fingernails and notice that wounds heal more slowly.

Diets that are too heavy in protein and do not contain enough carbohydrates can cause muscle wasting, low energy, constipation, bowel problems, liver and kidney problems, and gout.

Bread, cereals, rice, pasta and noodles

Grains and cereals can be found in a variety of products, including breakfast cereals – oats, muesli and wholegrain flakes – wholemeal breads and biscuits, rice, barley, corn and varieties of pasta.

Milk, yoghurt and cheese

Eat a diverse range of dairy foods including milk, yoghurt, cottage cheese and other types of cheese.

Breaking nutrition down into categories, in every meal you need to find a balance of carbohydrates, protein, fibre and micronutrients.

PUT A RAINBOW IN YOUR DIET

Different colours in fruit and vegetables indicate different 'phytonutrients'. This means, literally, the nutrients you get from plant foods. The more variety of natural colour you eat, the more likely it is that you are getting enough of these important nutrients.

As an exercise, think of the colours in your food on an average day. I asked a patient to do this recently. She is a very busy working mum who makes sure her three school-age children get the best possible diet to cover all their needs for growth and development. But she was forgetting to look after herself. The colours in her day looked like this:

- *Morning: porridge with brown sugar and a coffee with skim milk (beige and brown). At least she was eating breakfast.*

- *Morning tea: a few crackers with Vegemite and a cup of tea (beige and brown).*
- *Lunch: a chicken sandwich on white bread (beige and white).*
- *Dinner: whatever she had the energy to throw together. Usually, pasta.*

You get the message. Her food choices were leaving her with virtually no fruit and vegetables and she was feeling as colourless as her diet. So, think colour!

CARBOHYDRATES

If there is one dietary component that has an undeserved reputation, and grossly misunderstood and unfairly blamed, then it would have to be the carbohydrates. Just about every fad diet ever invented has demonised carbohydrates as the cause of everything from pimples to being overweight.

I often see patients looking for solutions to their problem with fatigue or trouble concentrating, and find that they are on a strict 'low-carb' diet. These diets can leave you feeling tired, dizzy, constipated, lethargic and fuzzy.

The problem is that you need carbohydrates for energy to carry out all of your body processes, including physical and mental activity and the functioning of your body organs. Of equal concern is that often these 'low-carb' diets are also low in fibre but high in animal fat.

What all carbohydrates have in common is that they provide glucose for the body's essential energy needs. Another important point is that there is a hierarchy of carbohydrates, from healthy to unhelpful.

The healthy sources of carbohydrates are whole grains, fruit and vegetables, and legumes. These foods come with stacks of vitamins, minerals and phytonutrients. So-called refined carbohydrates are the ones you need to steer away from. These are 'white foods' like white flour, white bread and refined sugar, which provide lots of kilojoules for little nutrient value. You do not need to eliminate these foods from your diet entirely; it is about balance. In general terms, you should include more fresh, unrefined and unprocessed wholefoods in your diet, and limit the highly refined and energy-dense but nutrient-poor foods.

❀ WHAT IS 'GI'?

You have probably heard the terms 'low GI' and 'high GI'. GI stands for 'glycaemic index'. This refers to the effect a carbohydrate food has on blood sugar levels, and does not refer to the amount of food you consume. Glycaemic load refers to the quantity of food you consume.

High GI foods are absorbed rapidly into the bloodstream, converted into glucose and increase blood glucose levels. Low GI foods take longer to absorb and cause a lower peak of blood sugar levels.

Bear in mind that the glycaemic index of a particular food refers to that food eaten on its own. As part of a balanced meal there is likely to be a combination of some low and some high GI foods. A healthy diet will emphasise a balance in favour of low GI rather than high GI foods.

A mainly low GI diet followed over many years has been shown to be associated with a lower risk of type 2 diabetes, coronary heart disease and age-related macular degeneration. A high GI diet is strongly associated with obesity.

❀ PROTEIN

Poorly balanced or fad diets often go wrong by having too much high-fat protein at the expense of fruit and vegetables, or too little protein. One of the groups I see who are most at risk in this regard are the vegetarians in families of omnivores. As with the scenario I described on page 135, one member of the family decides they don't want to eat meat any more, and they simply remove it from their serving of the family meals without making a concerted effort to replace the meat with another high-quality source of protein.

Protein deficiency is surprisingly common, particularly in vegetarians. Signs include muscle wasting and weakness, ankle swelling and anaemia.

On the flip side, very high protein diets are dangerous to your health because they often do not allow for enough carbohydrate to give you energy, or enough fibre to get your bowels moving normally. High protein diets can also increase the risk of liver and kidney problems, gout and gall bladder disease and, unless you increase calcium, as high protein increases kidney excretion of calcium, the long-term risk of osteoporosis.

Sources of protein

Proteins are made up of building blocks called amino acids. Essential amino acids have to be eaten as part of your diet. Animal sources of protein tend to have a balanced, complete set of amino acids. But with some knowledge and planning you can get enough protein from a vegetarian or vegan diet.

Animal sources

- *lean meat*
- *fish*
- *chicken and other poultry*
- *low-fat dairy products*
- *eggs.*

Vegetable sources

Proteins that come from vegetable sources tend to be low in one or more of the amino acids, so you will need to do some food-combining to get your daily protein needs:

- *legumes – beans, legumes, chick peas, soy products*
- *whole grains – rye, wheat, oats, rice, buckwheat, barley*
- *nuts and seeds*
- *tofu, tempeh and other soy products.*

Grains tend to be low in lysine, and legumes are low in methionine and tryptophan. By combining foods from different sources, you can make up all of your amino acid needs. For example, you can achieve this by combining legumes and grains, nuts and seeds with grains, or legumes with nuts and seeds to make up the right balance of amino acids to meet your protein needs if you do not eat animal-source proteins.

CAUTION WITH RED MEAT

We know that people who eat red meat – beef, veal, pork and lamb – have a higher risk of developing bowel cancer, heart disease and diabetes, and a higher risk of dying from heart disease, cancer, or for that matter, from any cause. Replacing red meat with fish, poultry, beans or nuts could help prevent heart disease and diabetes, and could lower the risk of early death. But doing that needs to be balanced against your need for vitamin B_{12} and iron. It is difficult to get enough of those nutrients without eating two to three serves of red meat a week.

Processed meat needs to be taken off the menu completely – bacon, hot dogs and meats such as salami – since they are known to further increase your risk of cancer, heart disease and diabetes.

🌿 OMEGA-3 ESSENTIAL FATTY ACIDS

There are three kinds of fatty acids: saturated, monounsaturated and polyunsaturated. Essential fatty acids (EFAs) are one group of the polyunsaturated fats. They are called 'essential' because they are essential to life, and have to be included in your diet because they cannot be made by your body and are not interchangeable.

The most important omega-3 EFAs are alpha-linoleic acid (ALA), eicosapentaenoic acid (EPA), and docosahexaenoic acid (DHA). Omega-3 is vital to all the cells in the body as a building block for the cell membrane. The membrane's job is to govern what goes in and out of the cell. Omega-3 supports the cell membrane's ability to control what goes in and out of the cell.

EFAs are particularly important components in the cell membranes of the brain, the retina of the eye and heart muscle. Researchers are looking into the role of omega-3 EFAs in health problems as diverse as diabetes, rheumatoid arthritis, ADHD, depression, certain cancers and cardiovascular disease, to name just a few.

EFAs have also been shown to lower triglyceride levels, make blood less likely to clot, decrease the growth rate of atherosclerotic plaque, or fat in the arteries, and lower blood pressure. These effects are important in reducing coronary heart disease as they keep the heart beating normally, reduce inflammation and support immune function.

Alpha-linolenic acid (ALA) is found in flaxseed and flaxseed oil, and in small quantities in walnuts, cold-pressed canola oil, wheat germ and dark green leafy vegetables. DHA and EPA are technically non-essential, because our bodies should be able to make these from ALA. They are considered 'essential', however, because in many people this conversion process does not happen efficiently if they don't get enough ALA in their diet, or vitamins C, B_6 and B_3, or zinc and magnesium, all of which are needed for the conversion. Eating too many omega-6 fats compared to omega-3, as is usually the case in Western diets, and elevated insulin levels, slows down the conversion. So most people need to get DHA and EPA from their diet.

The problem is that most Australians are not eating nearly enough omega-3 foods in their diets to maintain good health.

Omega-3 EFA food sources

By far the best food source of omega-3 EFAs is seafood, preferably oily fish such as sardines, salmon, swordfish, tuna and mackerel, as well as mussels, oysters and squid. Seafood contains both EPA and DHA.

But it seems that every silver lining has a cloud. With fish, it is mercury. Mercury content depends on factors such as the type of fish, its size, diet, age and habitat. The concentration increases the higher you go up the food chain to the larger predatory fish such as marlin, gemfish, orange roughy, swordfish, ray and shark. Food processing, preparation and cooking techniques do not significantly reduce the amount of mercury in fish. Fish with lower levels of mercury include mackerel, silver warehou, Atlantic salmon, canned salmon, herrings, tuna and sardines.

Fresh fish is the best source of omega-3, and plan for two to three meals a week of fish, using the type likely to have lower mercury content. There is a higher concentration of omega-3 in the skin of fish than in the flesh. You can buy seafood fresh, frozen, canned, dried, salted, smoked or processed.

Mercury exposure

The main concern regarding mercury exposure is for pregnant women because of the effect on neurological development of their unborn babies. Symptoms of mercury exposure include:

- impaired peripheral vision, hearing and speech
- disturbed sensation such as pins and needles in your hands and feet and around your mouth
- loss of coordination of movement
- muscle weakness.

Fresh fish caught and eaten within a day or two is ideal. Fish caught some distance away are frozen soon after they are caught and should be kept frozen until they are ready for preparation. The freshest seafood is available from outlets with a high turnover, such as fish markets or local seafood co-ops in fishing towns. Buy from shops that keep the seafood refrigerated and/or surrounded in ice at 0° to 1°C.

Supplements

Fish oil supplements have been shown to have so many health benefits that they are considered as a type of medication in some groups of people, particularly those with a history of heart disease, arthritis or depression. Omega-3 essential fatty acids deserve their 'buzz word' status, and the health benefits are a great reason to include seafood in your regular diet and to supplement if you cannot.

❧ FIBRE

Dietary fibre is found in all plant foods. We know from research that about 70 per cent of people do not eat enough vegetables, and almost 50 per cent do not eat enough fruit. Apart from all the nutrients they are missing out on, there is this other issue of fibre.

If you are feeling bloated or constipated and sluggish, you need to look at the amount of fibre in your diet. If you do not have enough fibre in your diet, and most people do not, it can contribute to constipation, irritable bowel syndrome, bowel cancer, cardiovascular disease, haemorrhoids and diverticulitis. Fibre also stabilises blood glucose and cholesterol levels.

There are two types of fibre: soluble and insoluble. Most whole foods contain some of both types.

Soluble fibre pulls in water to form a gel in the gut and softens faeces, making it easier to pass through your gut. Sources include fruit, vegetables, oat bran, barley, seed husks, flaxseed, psyllium husks, dried beans, lentils, peas and soy products.

Insoluble fibre acts as a natural laxative, which speeds up the transit of foods through the gut, bulks up stools and prevents constipation. Sources include wheat bran, corn bran, rice bran, fruit and vegetable skins, nuts, seeds and wholegrain foods.

If you have a low-fibre diet and decide to switch to a high-fibre diet, you might find your bowels object at first. If you increase fibre content suddenly, you can get flatulence and abdominal cramps. Introduce fibre gradually by increasing the amount of fruit and vegetables and other wholefoods into your diet.

MICRONUTRIENTS

You might hear a lot about the term 'micronutrients'. As their name suggests, they are the substances in your diet that you need in tiny amounts to maintain your body functions, metabolism and immunity. They are also known as vitamins and minerals. They are essential to your health and whether they are present in sufficient amounts to keep you healthy will depend on the quality and variety of foods you eat.

Micronutrient deficiencies are very common and cause health problems that can range from subtle to severe. For example, mild magnesium deficiency might show itself as muscular tics, leg cramps, muscle weakness and tiredness. More severe magnesium deficiency can cause low calcium and potassium levels, severe muscle spasms, loss of appetite, irritability, nausea, insulin resistance, irregular heartbeat and life-threatening heart failure.

Ideally, you will get all the micronutrients you need from a well-balanced, comprehensive and varied diet. Unfortunately this is a far too uncommon situation. Agricultural methods, food storage and cooking techniques, and your own gut's ability to absorb nutrients can all reduce the amount of micronutrient content that actually gets to your body cells.

DRINKING WATER

Hydration is such a simple concept: your body needs water for every single function in every cell. So, how much water is enough, and from what source?

One of the indicators of a developed country is the provision of plentiful safe drinking water to its population. Depending on where you live, your local water supply may be pure spring water, piped town water from a dam, bore water or water from a desalination plant.

There will be varying levels of minerals, suspended solids, bacteria and toxins in the water. Some supplies are considered safer than others. Some water supplies are deemed safe but have occasional incidents such as E. coli or Cryptosporidium or giardia contamination, enough to cause significant public health concerns. If you have any immune problems or you are concerned about the quality or consistency of your tap water, then you can have a high-quality water filter installed on your drinking water tap.

The amount of water you need varies depending on your size and your level of exertion, how hot the temperature is and the amount you sweat. Most of the water you drink will be in fluids like coffee, tea, juices, soft drinks, moisture in foods and of course water. If you drink lots of bottled water, remember that mineral water tends to contain sodium, which can cause fluid retention and ankle swelling, and can increase blood pressure. Make sure the drink bottles do not contain bisphenol-A, and consider the impact of plastic bottles on the environment.

There is not much point going through a list of every symptom you might have, from constipation to kidney stones, if you do not drink enough water. Every body function depends on water. You simply function better when you drink enough of it. Not enough, and you are dehydrated. And that can happen quite quickly.

A lot of people forget to drink, or underestimate the amount they need to drink in a day. I could say 'use your level of thirst as a guide', but some people mistake thirst for hunger and eat instead of having a drink of water.

As a starting point, you need to drink a minimum of six to eight 150 ml glasses of water a day. The requirement increases with special situations like exercising, air travel, breastfeeding and hot environments.

JUICES, SOFT DRINKS AND OTHER FLUIDS

Fluids count when you are assessing your diet. You need to consider how many soft drinks, fruit juices, and cappuccinos and other milky coffees you drink. A lot of people think that fruit juice is healthier than soft drink because it is full of 'natural' sugars. Fruit juice does contain natural sugar – fructose, sucrose and glucose – but the amount of sugar and kilojoules is on par with soft drinks. One fruit juice might contain the sugar equivalent of five or six pieces of fruit but without the fibre.

High-sugar-content drinks will stack on kilojoules and also cause a rapid increase in your blood fats, or triglycerides. If you are overweight, or have diabetes, or are carrying extra weight around the waist, you will need to control the amount of kilojoule-containing drinks you consume. Some US states and cities, including New York City, are starting campaigns to get tough on soft drinks and reduce consumption. Diet drinks containing artificial sweeteners are not a healthy alternative. They encourage sweet craving and lead to greater weight gain, not to mention the adverse effects some people experience with exposure to chemicals like aspartame.

PROCESSED FOODS

The way food is grown, harvested, stored, processed and cooked will affect its nutritional value. C and B group vitamins, particularly folate and thiamine, tend to be more unstable and destroyed by processing than the fat-soluble vitamins K, A, D and E.

Refining of grains reduces their nutrient quality. For example, if you remove the husks from cereals and grains during processing, you remove most of the fibre, B vitamins and other phytonutrients. That is why wholegrain breads and cereals are recommended for you instead of the more refined and processed foods.

Some nutrients are lost in the processes of freezing or canning, but the benefits of having more vegetables in your diet outweighs that loss. In general, focus on fresh, unprocessed or minimally processed foods where possible.

I should add here that cooking is a form of processing. Some foods lose their nutritional value when they are cooked. For example, peeling too much skin off can remove a lot of a vegetable's nutrients. But others need cooking to be edible or digestible, and to make them tastier. A few foods, like tomatoes, release greater nutritional value when they are cooked.

ORGANIC

There has been a phenomenal increase in interest in organic food across the Western world. The sale of organic food in China has quadrupled in the past five years, almost half of all baby food in the UK now sold is organic, and organic food is the fastest growing segment of food sales in many European countries. To a large extent, this movement has been consumer-led. The most often-cited reasons are concern over pesticides in conventionally produced food, desire for better food quality, animal welfare and environmental protection. The high-profile issues of mad cow disease and, more recently, avian influenza virus have also raised awareness about hazardous agricultural practices.

The term 'organic food' is usually taken to mean a food that has been produced without artificial fertilisers and that has not been treated with synthetic pesticides or growth promoters of any type, including hormones and antibiotics. It also refers to sustainable farming practices to return nutrients to the soil.

In general practice I am often asked whether it is worth the extra cost of buying organic. The question often comes about if someone is thinking about a detox, or if they have been feeling tired and lethargic, or after a diagnosis of illness such as cancer or multiple sclerosis where the patient feels they need to take control of their health in whatever way they can.

There is also an enormous amount of interest in organic food from parents of babies and young children concerned about the long-term effects of pesticide residues in conventional food. And rightly so. In recent US studies, blood samples of children aged two to four revealed concentrations of pesticides six times higher in children eating conventionally farmed fruit and vegetables compared with those eating organic food, and that reverting to an organic diet rapidly decreased the levels of pesticide residues.

Apart from the cancer-causing potential, exposure to agricultural pesticides has also been linked to hyperactivity, learning disabilities and behaviour disorders, memory problems and mood disorders.

> We know that pesticide residues in children drop rapidly when children are switched to a substantially organic diet.

On a broader scale, the issue is about finding a balance between high-yield agricultural practices aimed at providing volume of food year-round for entire populations, versus the health implications of poorer nutrient quality and possibly harmful additives in the food supply.

On a personal level, you need to decide whether you are prepared to pay the extra for organics to reduce your exposure to environmental chemicals. Availability is a key issue. Check your local area for stores or local growers' markets that stock organic products. It is a lot easier these days with the major supermarkets having an organic food section.

You may find it difficult to stay totally organic and still have wide variety in your food. Buy organic wherever you can and as much as you can to reduce your overall chemical exposure.

LOSING WEIGHT

If you are very obese, the task of reaching your healthy weight range may seem like too high a mountain to climb. But do not let that distant goal put you off. Even a relatively small weight loss, say, just 10 per cent of your current weight if you are overweight, will help to lower your risk of developing obesity-related diseases. A small but significant weight loss will also demonstrate to you that you can do it.

You may need to approach this in stages, setting progressive goals. Let's say that at 100 kg you are 30 kg over your healthy weight range. You might start with a goal of losing 10 per cent of your current weight, so getting to 90 kg is your initial goal. You may plateau at that weight to establish that you can easily sustain your program and then, with that success under your belt, set new goals with an accompanying eating plan and exercise program.

PLATEAUING

You may have had the experience of 'going on a diet', sticking rigidly to the formula and finding you lose weight for the first few weeks, just like the marketing brochures promised. Then you stop losing weight, and maybe even put on a few kilograms. This is the time when many people give up.

Before you embark on any substantial lifestyle change, you need to know to expect that there will be times, sometimes extended periods of time, when your progress seems to stall, your weight plateaus or you even put a kilo or two back on. This is a sign of physiological adjustment. If you can be patient and just maintain a holding pattern, your body chemistry will make the adjustment. At this point you will most likely need to make a change to your exercise plan, and increase and change some of your activities. Adding in weight training can be an effective strategy here. It may also signal that it is time for you to change your food intake as well.

Once you have had a medical check-up and a management plan put in place for any health conditions, you will need to have detailed information about an eating and activity plan that suits you.

Think about the types of activity that interest you (see the chapter 'Exercise', on page 171). Walking is a good way to start. You can also insert activity opportunities into your day. This might involve taking the stairs instead of the escalator, getting off the bus one stop early, or going for a stroll at lunchtime. If your excess weight makes it difficult for you to walk or run, then think of other ways to get moving, such as swimming, aqua-fitness, tai chi or a session on an exercise bike.

If you have a long-term weight problem, I would encourage you to see an accredited practicing dietitian to help you work out an eating plan you feel you can follow and one that accounts for all your nutritional and energy requirements. This needs to be a personalised plan, which takes into account your food preferences, family eating patterns, any cultural issues and your ability and willingness to prepare meals.

The reasons for being overweight can be quite simple problems with simple solutions. In my experience, though, sometimes there can be deep-seated psychological undercurrents that need to be sorted out before you can achieve long-term changes of entrenched eating behaviours. If you think there are psychological barriers to you making changes to your eating behaviour, it makes sense to talk to your doctor about a referral to a psychologist with expertise in this field.

The question of weight loss medication sometimes arises, although it comes up much less these days because the problems with adverse effects of these medications have been so well publicised. Over my years of clinical practice I have seen many of these drugs come and go, including fen-phen (fenfluramine and phentermine), ephedra, sibutramine and orlistat. They all have unacceptable risks or side effects.

I know it is tempting to think that there must be a quick fix to the problem of being overweight, but it really does need a strategic long-term plan and a lot of determination and persistence.

> The answers do not lie on a pharmacy shelf. The answers all lie within you.

ENERGY DENSITY

Most of the discussion around food has focused on fat content. While fat content is an important feature in weight control, it is not the only thing that matters. You also need to consider energy density.

Just because a food product is promoted as 'fat free' does not make it 'kilojoule free'. 'Fat free' food can still be loaded with sugar and carbohydrates.

As a general rule, increased fluid and fibre content will reduce the energy density, while highly processed food or food with a high content of carbs, fat or added sugar will tend to be more energy dense. Go for nutrient-dense foods with low energy density, not energy-dense foods with low nutrient density.

CASE STUDY

Sarah was in her 40s with two kids and a busy job. She had never really lost the weight she gained during her pregnancies. She was 162 cm tall and weighed 90 kg. Her BMI was 34. Her waist measurement was 100 cm. She never ate breakfast. The first time she ate in the day was at 11 am. She snacked throughout the afternoon and while preparing meals for the kids. She also had dinner with her husband each night after the kids' meal. She often drank half a bottle of wine with dinner during the week. She'd tried the Paleo diet, the Dukan diet, the South Beach diet, the Atkins diet but none had worked. First I got her to keep a food diary, then I sent her to a dietician who worked out a structured eating plan for her. She was to eat three meals and two small snacks a day. The plan had the right balance of protein and carbs with plenty of vegies. She cut down on alcohol; drinking no more than two glasses three times a week. She also got off the bus a stop earlier to walk home. After two weeks, she was disappointed that she had only lost 1 kg. I explained that .5 kg weight loss per week was exactly the right amount. It would be sustainable for her in the long run. Over the next 60 weeks, she lost 30 kilos. She said it was so easy that she hardly even noticed she was on an eating plan. So far, she has stayed with the plan and kept her weight at the same healthy level.

PORTION SIZE

If you are overweight or underweight, the matter of portion size inevitably needs to be addressed. Portion size is, literally, the quantity of food you eat.

I will tell you about one common scenario I see in my practice. A woman with an obesity problem is asking for advice on how to get down to her healthy weight range. She eats 'just like everyone else in the family' but cannot seem to get her weight down.

The next obvious question is, 'Who lives at home with you?' This question is important because it logically follows that whoever lives at home with you will have a big influence on what you eat and how much.

Consider the case of a woman who is 155 cm tall, lives with her husband and two adult sons who are all big men with large frames and stand about

185 cm tall. Now think about 'plating up' at dinnertime. Almost invariably, all the meals will be plated up the same portion size. Now think about each person's kilojoule requirements. If they all eat more or less the same quantity of food, guess who is going to be overweight. Of course it will be the woman, who is much shorter and has lower kilojoule requirements than the men.

Given the epidemic of being overweight and obesity in the developed world, there is no question that the issue of too-large portion sizes is a big problem. And it seems that everything is conspiring to create the impression that huge portion sizes are the norm. The fashion of dinner plates the size of a satellite dish and drinking glasses the size of a goldfish bowl would be one factor.

One simple technique to reduce portion sizes is to use smaller plates. The plate looks full, but it takes less food to make it look full.

One of the difficulties with controlling portion size is that if you eat out a lot or buy takeaway, the portion sizes are controlled by the food retailer. There has been a competition between food outlets for bigger servings for the same price or a relatively small price increase, creating the impression of better 'value'. If all the competing outlets serve are burgers and chips, then the only point of comparison is the size of the serving.

Reducing portion sizes

- Use a small-size dinner plate.
- Stop eating when you are no longer hungry.
- If you order pasta when you are at a restaurant, choose the appetiser size.
- In restaurants with large portion sizes, order two appetisers instead of an appetiser and a main meal.
- When buying packaged food from the supermarket, choose smaller packet sizes.
- If you order fries with a meal, share them. Better still, order green vegetables as a side dish.
- Avoid 'all you can eat' buffets.

After buying the food, the tendency is to finish the meal rather than throw some of it away once you have eaten enough to satisfy your needs.

We rarely, if ever, actually measure or weigh our food, so it comes down to a 'best guess' about how much food to prepare and serve.

When I point out the appropriate serving size or portion size to a patient, the reaction is usually one of surprise. One example is when I explain that the recommended portion size for a steak is the palm of your hand, not including your fingers, or the size of a deck of cards. That should be about one-quarter of the plate, with another quarter occupied by a carbohydrate and the remaining half with non-starchy vegetables.

ALL ABOUT BALANCE

Harvard Medical School developed a Healthy Eating Plate to illustrate the most appropriate balance of nutrients for your diet:

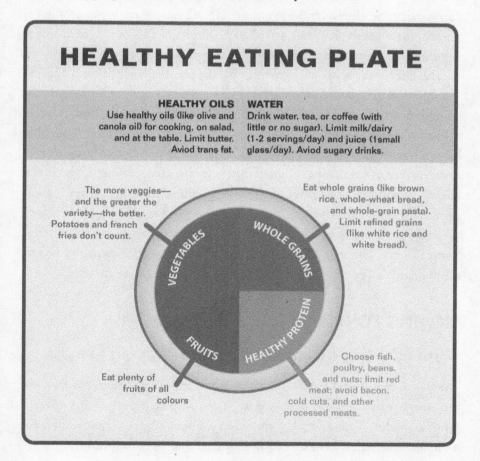

HEALTHY EATING PLATE

HEALTHY OILS
Use healthy oils (like olive and canola oil) for cooking, on salad, and at the table. Limit butter. Avoid trans fat.

WATER
Drink water, tea, or coffee (with little or no sugar). Limit milk/dairy (1-2 servings/day) and juice (1 small glass/day). Aviod sugary drinks.

The more veggies—and the greater the variety—the better. Potatoes and french fries don't count.

VEGETABLES

Eat whole grains (like brown rice, whole-wheat bread, and whole-grain pasta). Limit refined grains (like white rice and white bread).

WHOLE GRAINS

FRUITS

HEALTHY PROTEIN

Eat plenty of fruits of all colours

Choose fish, poultry, beans, and nuts; limit red meat; avoid bacon, cold cuts, and other processed meats.

SPECIAL NEEDS

Not everyone is the same when it comes to being able to tolerate food of every type. Food intolerance is a term that is thrown around a lot, but it can be a massive problem if you have a food intolerance that has not been diagnosed, or if you are exposed to a food you should not be eating.

I talk about that more in the chapter 'Food Intolerance and Food Allergy', on page 165.

SUPPLEMENTS (SEE CHAPTER ON VITAMINS AND SUPPLEMENTS)

The mantra you often hear that 'you can get all you need from food' is overly simplistic and does not hold true for many people in the community, particularly the elderly and the chronically ill, people with gut problems, vegans, fussy eaters, adolescents, alcohol-imbibers and pregnant women. Actually, that doesn't leave too many of us.

This fact was recognised recently by the Australian National Health and Medical Research Council (NHMRC) when it revised its nutritional guidelines for the first time since 1991, acknowledging that different levels apply for avoiding nutrient deficiency, preventing chronic illness such as heart disease and some cancers, and for different population groups. But nutrition is not just about minimal nutrient quantities. It is also about the quality of food production and processing, the availability of fresh food depending on where you live, and preparation and cooking techniques.

I go into a lot more detail in the chapter 'Vitamins and Nutritional Supplements', on page 253, looking at deficiencies and when you need to supplement as specific therapy for particular medical conditions.

MOVING FORWARD

YOUR NEW EATING PLAN FOR LIFELONG GOOD HEALTH

There is no point 'going on a diet', certainly not permanently. That fits into the category of cruel and unreasonable punishment, especially if you are a bit of a 'foodie'. Sound, healthy nutrition is about ensuring that you create a lifelong pattern of healthy eating that becomes your new normal.

You can tailor a new individual eating plan that satisfies your hunger, your energy needs, your food tastes, your social life and any special health needs. You can also allow yourself a bit of freedom for special events.

Your new normal eating plan will need to consider all of the principles we have discussed:

- *Shop for fresh food regularly*
- *Eat breakfast*
- *Plan healthy lunches*
- *Have a range of simple recipes*
- *Eat a rainbow*
- *Include 2 pieces of fruit a day*
- *Include 5 serves of vegetables a day*
- *Remember to balance protein and carbohydrates*
- *Control quantity and quality of snacking*
- *Remember omega-3 (fish)*
- *Supplement where necessary.*

GOALS

Here are a few suggestions from me as to what goals you might set for yourself regarding your diet:

- *To complete an accurate food diary for one week*
- *To eat breakfast every day*
- *To have a healthy BMI*
- *To have a waist measurement in the healthy range.*
- *To follow the principles of 'mindful eating'*
- *To make a plan for lunch and dinner every day*
- *To make a plan for regular fresh food shopping and stocking of my pantry*
- *To eliminate preservatives, artificial colourings and flavourings, and processed and packaged foods as much as possible from my diet*
- *To follow the principles of a healthy balanced diet*
- *To make sure there are two serves of fruit and five serves of vegetables in my diet every day*
- *To check for sources of protein, iron, and essential vitamins and minerals in my diet*
- *To see a dietician if I am not sure about the nutritional quality of my diet.*

YOUR GOALS

Goal	Action	Obstacles/solution	Result
Eat breakfast	Buy cereal and milk on the weekend	Being too busy: be more organised	More energy throughout the day

FOOD INTOLERANCE AND FOOD ALLERGY

If you want to work out why you are not feeling your best, we need to look at whether you might have a problem with something you are eating. In the chapter on nutrition, we looked at the amount and quality of the food you are eating. A related but quite different issue is the possibility that something you are eating does not agree with your body chemistry. That can create a number of reactions, including food intolerance and food allergy, which are different things.

How do you know if you might have an allergy or intolerance to food?

SYMPTOMS OF FOOD ALLERGY

After eating particular foods:

- *swelling, itching or burning in and around the mouth*
- *skin rash, hives*
- *nausea and vomiting*
- *diarrhoea, abdominal pains*
- *trouble breathing, sometimes life-threatening.*

SYMPTOMS OF FOOD INTOLERANCE

After eating particular foods:

- *fatigue*
- *feeling 'just not right'*
- *irritable bowel symptoms – constipation, diarrhoea, gripey abdominal pains, gas*
- *anxiety*
- *sweating*
- *headaches*
- *breathing problems*
- *palpitations*
- *trouble sleeping.*

There is a lot of crossover between the symptoms of food intolerance and food allergy. To tell the difference you need to have specialised medical testing.

You can have an intolerance to a food, to components of a food, or to the additives or chemicals added to a food. There are many types of food intolerance, but I will concentrate on the two most common types: gluten and lactose.

LACTOSE INTOLERANCE

Lactose intolerance is when you are unable to digest dairy products containing lactose. This can occur in anyone, but it is more common in people with ethnic background from Asia, the Middle East and some Mediterranean countries.

You might be born with permanent lactose intolerance (from a deficiency of the enzyme lactase in your gut), or it can develop later. Sometimes you can develop a transient form of lactose intolerance after a gut infection.

If you have lactose intolerance and you eat or drink anything containing lactose, you might get excess gas, abdominal pains, bloating and diarrhoea. Avoiding lactose may take some changes to your diet but you should be able to adapt without too much trouble. Look for lactose-free products.

GLUTEN INTOLERANCE

It is not until someone suggests to you that your health problems might be fixed if you eliminated gluten from your diet that you realise how heavily most Western diets rely on it. Today it is far easier to go gluten free than it was even just a few years go, but there are still pitfalls and hidden gluten in many foods.

Gluten is in wheat, oats, rye, barley, triticale and thickeners.

Most people in the population tolerate gluten in their diets with no apparent problem, but if you have gluten intolerance, going gluten free is the best thing that can happen to you. Gluten intolerance takes many forms and has physical and emotional effects. It is really important that you don't think about gluten intolerance as a problem only with the gut.

This is a problem that can affect the whole body, every organ, your mood and personality and it can impact on your work, friendships and family relationships.

Gluten sensitivity is still not taken as seriously as it needs to be: by the medical profession, the food industry and the general public, many of whom are largely unaware of the potential dangers of gluten exposure for some people.

The diagnosis of a food intolerance can be a mixed blessing. On the one hand there is sadness and frustration that foods others can happily enjoy are quite possibly out of your life forever. On the other hand, such a diagnosis could be the best thing that ever happened to you because it could be the explanation for why you have been feeling so bad, and guides you to a diet that can have you feeling well and full of energy again.

Reactions to a diagnosis of food intolerance:

- *grief*
- *frustration*
- *sense of isolation*
- *stress and anxiety*
- *depression*
- *fear of accidental exposure*
- *mistrust*
- *reduced health-related quality of life*
- *disruption to family activities.*

Gluten intolerance can take may forms:

- *abdominal bloating, abdominal pain, occasional diarrhoea, indigestion*
- *trouble getting pregnant*
- *behavioural and learning problems in children*
- *clumsiness, gluten headaches, 'brain fog'*
- *tiredness*
- *depression, anxiety, irritability*
- *skin rash.*

Hidden sources of gluten include:

- *some medications and vitamins*
- *food preparation techniques in restaurants – tossing 'grilled' fish in flour lining soufflé dishes with flour*
- *packaged stock*
- *soy sauce*
- *basting sauces*
- *'cornflour' that isn't – some cornflours are wheaten cornflour*
- *French fries and hash browns – commercially prepared French fries, as opposed to hand cut, are tossed in flour for freezing and storage*
- *some salad dressings use gluten in thickeners*
- *soups and sauces*
- *some tea bags*
- *communion wafers.*

MANAGING GLUTEN INTOLERANCE

Knowing the harm that gluten can cause you if you are sensitive to it, you will be glad to be gluten free. Educate yourself, your family and your friends about the obvious and hidden sources of gluten: stock cubes, soups, gravy mixes, Vegemite, sauces, floured fish, malt on cornflakes (see the list above).

Buy a collection of gluten-free cookbooks and recipes. Do a fact-finding trip to the supermarket to check out their gluten-free section to replace your usual gluten-containing foods. And taste-test some of the alternatives to gluten-containing products.

EATING OUT

Call ahead to a restaurant to make sure it accommodates special diets without making you feel like a freak, and be assertive with waiters. You really need to insist that they pay attention to your food allergies. Most reasonable restaurants are aware of their moral and legal responsibility to customers with a food allergy or intolerance, and are able to work around their existing menu or amend dishes to suit you. Some even have special gluten-free menu cards.

If you are invited to share a meal with a friend or family member, make sure they understand how important it is for you to know what is in each dish. If you are in doubt, don't eat it. I know some people with food intolerances who actually take a contingency pack of food in case they turn up to an event where the food is particularly unfriendly to them.

> Knowing about gluten intolerance is more than halfway to dealing with it.

The best way to treat food intolerance is to isolate the food that is causing problems and eliminate it from your diet completely. This should be done with the supervision and advice of a dietitian.

If you know you have a food intolerance, don't be pressured by anyone into eating something you don't tolerate, because you can feel awful for days or even weeks afterwards.

> FODMAP stands for Fermentable Oligo-, Di-, Mono-saccharides And Polyols which are food components that cause the bowel to distend and thereby produce symptoms of excessive wind, bloating and cramps. It is often the case that a patient with, say, a wheat intolerance will also show symptoms of other food intolerances, such as lactose intolerance or fructose malabsorption. The consumption of a variety of high-FODMAP foods has a cumulative effect, increasing the severity of symptoms. Australian researchers have developed a low-FODMAP diet, which is fast becoming a catchall approach for those suffering from one or more intolerances. If you have a sensitive dietary system and you are finding it difficult to work out which food groups trigger particular symptoms, a low-FODMAP diet could be the solution. Most dieticians and nutritionists are now aware of this approach and will be able to design a low-FODMAP plan for you.

MOVING FORWARD

If you suspect you may have a food allergy or food intolerance, make an appointment to see your GP and get the appropriate medical tests. You may have to make significant changes to your diet and lifestyle but the sooner you do, the sooner you will feel a whole lot better.

YOUR GOALS

Goal	Action	Obstacles/solutions	Result
Diagnose and treat suspected food intolerance	Go to my GP and be tested	More difficulty in eating foods: plan my meals more carefully	Feel great! Much healthier

EXERCISE

When I am taking a medical history, one of the key questions I ask patients is what sort of exercise they do, at what intensity and how often. It is amazing the number of people who feel below par, yet they neglect this most basic function of their bodies: movement. They are surprised if they get puffed going up a flight of stairs or carrying the shopping in from the car, when that is the only time they are moving at all. And they wonder why they don't have the energy reserves to do the things they would like to do. There is usually no shortage of good intentions, but paying for a gym membership that is never used is not the same as committing to regular activity.

Whether you were a child sports star or one of those kids who faked illness to get out of PE classes, exercise, or at least some form of physical activity, is an essential ingredient in any path to optimal health. The aim of exercise is to improve or maintain your body's form and function, to help you relax, and hopefully you will actually enjoy it.

You don't have to be an elite athlete. The great thing about exercise for the sake of your health is that you have so much choice, and you can find an appropriate type of exercise to suit your preferences and the outcome you want to achieve. You can join a team, like the local netball or soccer team or a social tennis group, a golf club or a bushwalking group. You might prefer to go it alone with regular walks, swimming, surfing, gardening or gym-based fitness training. You could take individual or group classes in yoga, Pilates or tai chi.

At every opportunity throughout the day, you can take exercise opportunities such as walking up the stairs instead of taking the escalator, walking to the local shops instead of taking the car, or cycling to work.

WHY EXERCISE?

The human body evolved with movement in mind. Our physical structure and our bodies' metabolic and biochemical functions are geared to a level of activity that few people in modern life actually do. With the rise in technology, the trend to a more sedentary lifestyle has risen in parallel. Instead of exercise being an integral part of everyday survival, it has to be consciously factored into your day.

Let's look at the main reasons why it is important to get yourself moving:

- **Exercise increases your energy**. *Do it right, and expending energy actually gives you energy. Sound weird? Think of it like this. Fitness is about efficiency. Exercise increases muscle strength and improves heart and lung function. The improved delivery of oxygen and other essential nutrients to every cell in your body in turn helps those body cells to perform their essential functions more efficiently, improving energy production.*

- **Exercise helps you to sleep better**. *Being active during the day and exercising regularly improves sleep quality at night and wakefulness in the day. Try to avoid exercising vigorously too close to bedtime because it activates your sympathetic nervous system (SNS) and increases your alertness, making it more difficult to get to sleep. It is better to exercise earlier in the day or to have a period of quiet activity between exercising and when you go to bed. Many medical conditions cause tiredness and fatigue, regardless of the amount of sleep you get. But if you are otherwise in reasonable health, oversleeping can make you feel chronically tired. Rather than getting more sleep to raise your energy level, often what is needed is more activity in your day and setting an alarm so you don't sleep past what your body and mind actually need.*

- **Exercise makes you happier.** *We know that exercise is an effective part of the treatment for anyone with anxiety and/or depression at any age. That being said, because lack of motivation is a feature of some types of depression, it can be a challenge to start and maintain a regular schedule of exercise. You can get extra motivation by organising to meet up with a friend for a walk or a swim. To be effective, exercise has to be regular. That doesn't mean once a year on your birthday but every day, regardless of the weather, or your mood, or whatever other things might come up as excuses. You can see mood elevation at any age with pretty much any form of exercise, but aerobic – huff and puff – exercise appears to be most effective in improving mental health. Higher-intensity exercise seems to be more effective than low-intensity exercise. You get an immediate effect during the exercise session, but you will experience sustained improvement with a sustained exercise habit. There are a number of explanations for this, including the release of endorphins, the calming effect of an increase in body temperature, improved blood circulation in the brain, and the impact on the hypothalamic–pituitary–adrenal axis modifying the physiological reaction to stress. It might also have* *something to do with distraction from worries and improved self-esteem. Exercise also helps to manage alcohol and substance abuse, which are often forms of self-medication for people with mental health issues.*

Why exercise makes you happier

- improves your general health, physical fitness and sense of wellbeing
- improves sleep
- makes you feel better about yourself through a sense of achievement
- distracts you from problems, temporarily providing relief from worries
- helps release negative or destructive emotions such as anger, hostility and frustration
- enables greater social engagement, especially in shared activities or team/club sports
- increases cerebral neurotransmitters, such as serotonin
- reduces the need for medications used to manage symptoms of depression and anxiety

---

- **Exercise improves your health**, *whatever state of health you are in. It can even cure disease. Along with poor nutrition and tobacco use, lack of exercise is one of the top three risk factors for chronic disease.*

- **Exercise helps control your weight.** *Energy expended is energy that does not get stored as body fat.*

- **Exercise is good for your sex life.** *I deliberately tacked this on the end to give you an extra incentive, but it's true. I could go on about endurance and flexibility, but I'm sure you get the picture.*

EXERCISE AND DISEASE

CARDIOVASCULAR DISEASE

Regular exercise provides a strong protection against cardiovascular disease. This is because of the effects of exercise in reducing heart disease risk factors. Exercise:

- *reduces body fat*

- *helps you achieve and maintain healthy body weight*
- *improves cholesterol and triglycerides, or blood fats*
- *reduces blood pressure*
- *increases efficient heart and blood vessel function.*

Exercise is an integral part of the recovery and rehabilitation from heart attack or stroke. A combination of aerobic and anabolic or resistance exercise is recommended, and has been shown to significantly improve longevity and quality of life.

❧ OSTEOARTHRITIS

Osteoarthritis is one of the most common causes of pain and disability in older adults. Some forms of activity will be painful, but reducing activity will exacerbate the disease. Exercise, in particular strength training, can reduce joint stiffness and strengthen the muscles supporting affected joints. Exercise also improves your ability to do daily activities like walking, going up and down stairs, and getting up from a chair.

❧ CANCER

If you have been diagnosed with cancer there is a lot of focus on treating cancer with surgery, radiotherapy and chemotherapy. What we are starting to hear more about is how to go beyond basic recovery from the illness, to feeling even better than you did before your diagnosis. We now recognise the importance of maintaining an appropriate form of exercise throughout the treatment process as an integral part of cancer treatment.

After a diagnosis of cancer, regular exercise will improve the outcome of surgery, reduce symptoms and help manage the side effects of chemotherapy and radiotherapy. It also helps to maintain your physical functioning and reduce the likelihood of muscle wasting and bone loss that come with prolonged inactivity. A compelling argument for exercise after a diagnosis of cancers, such as breast and colorectal, is that it significantly increases survival.

❧ OSTEOPOROSIS

Competitive sport in childhood has been shown to result in higher bone density in older age. The activity needs to be ground-based and with higher loads and impacts. For example, bone mineral density in weightlifters is higher than other active people, and this continues into later life. Swimming, however, does not have a protective effect on bone.

Physical activity in later life can improve or at least slow bone loss as you get older, and the most effective form of exercise appears to be anabolic, or resistance, exercise.

❧ IMMUNITY

An impaired immune system weakens the body's ability to fight off infection and malignancy. There are a number of ways to boost your immune system, and that includes regular exercise. Research studies have shown that regular brisk walking can bolster many defences of the immune system, including the antibody response and the natural killer, or T cell, response. See the chapter, 'Immunity', on page 188, for more information.

> Your immune system needs lower intensity and shorter duration of exercise than you need for cardiovascular training. About 20 to 30 minutes of brisk walking five days per week will maintain a healthy immune response.

❧ FIGHTING THE EFFECTS OF AGEING

As you get older, it is easy to explain away a general sense of fatigue or your loss of strength and fitness as the inevitable signs of age. But the difference between a frail and physically vulnerable older person and one who is active and involved in life to their maximum potential often comes down to a long-term exercise strategy.

We also know that lifelong physical activity can delay the onset of Alzheimer's even in those with a high genetic predisposition. In the early stages, regular exercise slows the progression of the disease, helping to maintain both physical and cognitive capacity. Even a single episode of exercise results in short-term improvement in memory and brain function in patients with existing dementia.

Exercise also prevents and reverses muscle loss in the elderly, and reduces the likelihood of falls and fractures.

Think you're too old to start? Consider that increases in life expectancy are possible even in people who do not begin regular exercise until age 75.

Snapshot of the problem

* Rate of sedentary and low exercise levels: 70 per cent of Australians over 15 years of age.
* Females (73 per cent) are more sedentary than males (66 per cent).
* Over 75 years of age the rate increases to a worrying 83 per cent.
* The rate is lowest in the 15–24-year-old group, but still comes in at 62 per cent!
* Children are more likely to reach activity targets.
* Internationally, the data are similar for other developed nations.
* Physical activity levels appear to be decreasing markedly in developing countries.

WHAT EXERCISE CAN DO FOR YOU

AEROBIC EXERCISE

Aerobic exercise is the sort of activity that makes you sweat and puff. Using the large muscle groups, it might involve walking, cycling, swimming, dancing, running or rowing. Ideally, it is performed at low to moderate intensity over a long period of time.

You can also accumulate bouts of exercise; for example, a brisk 10-minute walk three times a day.

Benefits of aerobic exercise:

* *reduces systolic and diastolic hypertension*
* *improves heart function*
* *improves respiratory function*
* *increases stamina*
* *increases muscle strength and function*

- *increases haemoglobin – iron-carrying protein in red blood cells*
- *activates your immune system*
- *reduces blood lipids – LDL, or 'bad' cholesterol and triglycerides*
- *reduces the risk of chronic diseases such as diabetes, heart disease, obesity and hypertension*
- *increases HDL – 'good' cholesterol*
- *reduces body fat*
- *improves glucose metabolism*
- *maintains or increases bone density and reduces fracture risk, increasing the chance for independence in old age*
- *makes you feel happier*
- *reduces cognitive decline in older age*
- *improves quality of life.*

Recommended rates of aerobic exercise

- ❧ Do moderately intense cardio 30 minutes a day, 5 days a week, OR
- ❧ do vigorously intense cardio 20 minutes a day, 3 days a week, OR
- ❧ a combination of moderate and vigorous sessions.

❧ RESISTANCE TRAINING

Resistance training is characterised by short intense bursts of movement against the resistance of weights, elastic or resistance machines. The amount of resistance is set so that the number of repetitions you are physically able to do in each set of exercises is 12 or fewer.

Recommended resistance levels

Do 8–10 different strength-training exercises, 8–12 repetitions of each exercise, repeated 3–4 times, at least twice a week.

If you are able to do more than 12 repetitions in a set, the amount of resistance needs to be increased to get the positive effects of strengthening your muscles, building your bones and releasing hormones. To achieve the desired effect, the resistance program needs to be done regularly, two to three times a week.

Benefits of resistance training:

- *reduces body fat*
- *increases muscle strength*
- *improves balance*
- *reduces risk of falls*
- *maintains or increases bone density*
- *makes you happier*
- *improves quality of life.*

If you want to further improve your physical fitness, reduce your risk of chronic disease and disability and prevent weight gain or lose weight, you can exceed these minimum targets according to your ability.

Flexibility

Lack of flexibility is a common problem for people who lead a sedentary lifestyle, and it gets worse as you grow older. Flexibility naturally decreases with age unless you actively work to maintain it. On the whole, women tend to be more flexible than men at all ages.

Flexibility is a term that refers to the total range of motion of a joint, or group of joints. The degree of flexibility depends on the structure of the joint and the mechanics of the muscles and soft tissues around the joint. Holding a muscle in a position that places it on stretch and repeating over time causes the muscle to increase in length, which in turn increases the range of motion of the joint.

Benefits of flexibility training:

- *reduces muscle soreness after exercise*
- *improves posture*
- *reduces injury*
- *reduces lower back pain*
- *increases functional range of motion*
- *delays muscle fatigue*
- *helps relaxation.*

The goal of flexibility training is to optimise joint mobility while maintaining joint stability.

SO, WHAT'S STOPPING YOU?

If your exercise diary has shown you that you are not exercising enough – or at all! – then you should definitely consider changing your habits and making exercise a priority. One of the hardest things about changing entrenched habits, especially bad ones, is getting a start. If you have not done a scrap of exercise since you were in primary school, then you need to think about what you might enjoy doing. There is no point signing up for aqua fitness if you don't like getting your hair wet. You might need to try a few different types of activity before you find one or two that you enjoy.

Talk to your friends about the activities they do to see if there is something that takes your interest. Perhaps one of your friends or a family member will go along with you to give you some initial encouragement.

Getting a start can be a bit overwhelming if you don't know where to go, what to expect, don't know what gear you need, how to use it and whether you are likely to do yourself any damage in the process. Proper form and instruction will reduce the chance of injuries so take lessons, even if you are not a complete beginner to a sport.

Some people do not like the unfamiliar physical sensation of sweating or increased heart rate or muscular exertion, or the aching muscles the next day if they overdo it. If that is you, then you will just have to take my word for it that the positive effects of exercise on your body and mind will have you actually enjoying the physical sensations that accompany a good workout. Eventually.

You need an initial motivator, a spark that ignites you to take on a different pattern of behaviour. A lot of the time in medical practice, I see the 'spark' coming in the form of a major health scare. There is nothing like a potentially life-threatening diagnosis to focus your attention on your health as a priority.

Many years back when I faced my own personal medical crisis, my specialist at the time sat on the hospital bed and said to me, 'Whatever you do from now on, you must exercise an hour every day, no matter what.

That is a priority above all else.' I believed him. I tell my patients the same thing. Put it in your diary in the same way as any important event in your day, and work around it. If you don't make exercise a priority, something will come along to make it a priority for you.

❧ FINDING THE TIME

Finding the time is one of the big excuses people use to put off getting fit. Making exercise a priority will sort out any time issues. Ideally, set the alarm a bit earlier in the morning and get your exercise out of the way before you go to work. If that is impossible, then take your walking shoes or gym gear to work and fit in exercise in the middle of the day. Even a half-hour walk at lunchtime will give you benefits.

There is a concept we call 'incidental exercise', which almost makes it sound like an accident. It means using opportunities for activity during your waking hours to accumulate as many minutes each day of non-sedentary time as you can, and in particular to reduce the time spent sitting. I know a psychotherapist who finds it very effective to have 'walk and talk' sessions with his clients. I have a friend who has a business in the city and asks clients to meet him in their walking gear to walk while they discuss business deals. You can walk from the railway station to work instead of getting a taxi or bus. You can walk to the local shops instead of taking your car. Or take the stairs rather than the lift. You will find that physical activity improves your overall work efficiency.

> Remember, the total minimum time commitment required is only 150 minutes of aerobic exercise and 90 minutes of strength training per week. *Just over half an hour per day.*

❧ SAFETY FIRST

If you are over 35 and you have any medical problems or risk factors for heart disease such as smoking or high blood pressure, then it is wise to see your doctor for a pre-activity check-up. If you have had a medical problem and you are concerned about starting to exercise because you don't know how much or what to do, talk to your GP about the type of exercise that might be suitable for you.

Case Study

Jeff was a star front row forward during High School. When he went to uni, he gained 15 kg in the first year alone. He then went into a career in the corporate sector. A routine check-up, prompted by his wife, just before his fortieth birthday revealed his BMI was 36. His risk of heart disease was very high, he was doing no exercise and drinking an average of twenty drinks a week. He admitted that about five years ago he'd gone for a run and been so sore afterwards he couldn't move for a week. In addition to a change in diet and cutting down on alcohol, I suggested he get the running shoes back out and start walking 45 minutes a day, just to the point of being puffed. After a while he incorporated some hills into his walk and picked the pace further. Three months later, he'd lost 12 kg, his sleep was better, he felt happier and he swore he'd never let himself get so unhealthy again.

You could have a qualified exercise professional set up a program for you. This would be a personal trainer, an exercise physiologist, a rehabilitation expert or a physiotherapist.

One of the main mistakes I see people making is to go too hard when they are unfit and just starting out, or deciding to get fit again when they haven't done anything more active for years than bending down to tie their shoelaces. Getting exhausted or injured in the early phases of your fitness program will discourage you. So if you are going to do your own thing unsupervised, it is important to start slowly and build up time and intensity gradually as your fitness improves.

Regardless of any illness or injury, there will be the potential to perform some form of physical activity to improve your health and a practical strategy to overcome any barrier.

HOW TO PLAN AN EXERCISE SESSION

❧ WARMING UP

'Warming up' refers to five to 10 minutes of activity at the start of an exercise session. The aim of this low-intensity aerobic movement is to increase the blood flow to muscles and tendons and to gradually increase the heart's pumping rate. Warming up reduces the risk of injury and cardiovascular events and prepares your body for more intense activity. For example, if you are going for a run, you don't start with a sprint. You start with a walk, increasing to a brisk pace, before breaking into a running pace.

🌿 AEROBIC EXERCISE

You can gauge the intensity of your exercise by how you are feeling. As a rough guide, when you are starting out aim for feeling slightly out of breath and warm. The rise in your heart rate will depend on the intensity of your activity, your age and your general fitness.

For those who like to be able to put a number to the target heart rate, the simplest measure of the intensity of aerobic or cardiorespiratory training is 20–60 minutes of continuous or intermittent aerobic activity training at 60–90 per cent of your maximum heart rate, or MaxHR.

> EXAMPLE: If you are 50 years old, your maxHR is 170 beats per minute.
> Your target training heart rate at 60–90 per cent of the maxHR is in the range of 102–153 beats per minute.

The simplest method for measuring heart rate is to count your pulse at the wrist for 15 seconds and then multiply that by four to calculate beats per minute. Alternatively, you can buy an electronic heart-rate monitor from any sports store. The advantage of monitoring your heart rate during exercise sessions is to make sure you are reaching an adequate intensity but not overdoing it.

🌿 RESISTANCE TRAINING

The basic unit of a resistance training session is the repetition. For a specific exercise, a repetition is the completion of one cycle, from the starting position through the end of the movement and back to the start. In strength training, a series of eight to 12 repetitions is normally completed and this is termed a 'set'.

Towards the end of the set your muscles will start to fatigue, and performing the exercise will become more difficult. By the end of the repetitions, you should not be able to do any more repetitions. Wait until your muscles recover and then repeat the exercise. The period between sets is called 'rest' or 'recovery'.

When you are planning anabolic or resistance exercises there are some general rules:

- *Do 8–10 different strength-training exercises, with three to four sets of 8–12 repetitions of each exercise, at least twice a week.*
- *As your muscle strength increases you will need to increase the load or resistance to increase the effect.*
- *Exercise large muscle groups first (for example, leg squats).*
- *Do the multi-joint exercises like bench presses or lunges before the more specific single-joint exercises (for example, biceps curls).*
- *Do your abdominal and lower-back exercises after whole-body ground-based exercises such as squats, dead lifts, bench presses and so on, to avoid fatiguing the muscle groups that stabilise and support the trunk and spine.*
- *Do not leave abdominal and lower-back exercises until the end, in case you don't get around to doing them. These exercises are very important for posture and protecting the lower back, and they have to be completed during each session.*

❧ COOL-DOWN AND STRETCH

The cool-down allows your cardiovascular system to gradually adjust to resting levels after a period of intense activity. It will prevent dizziness, which might happen as a result of blood pooling in your warmed-up leg muscles if you stop exercise suddenly.

It allows your muscles to gradually cool down, dissipates lactic acid build-up in muscles and prepares you to stretch your main muscle groups.

> For an effective cool-down perform low-intensity exercise for a minimum of five to 10 minutes and follow this with a stretching routine.

Expert advice on a safe and effective exercise program is an excellent investment, because it will improve your confidence and ensure you are on the right track.

OVERWEIGHT AND OBESITY

If you are overweight, reducing your weight by just 10 per cent can decrease your blood pressure, lower your blood cholesterol level and reduce your risk of diabetes. The solution comes down to a formula of less energy or kilojoules in, more energy out. In other words: less food plus more activity.

If you are losing weight you need to be doing exercise to make sure muscles and bone density are maintained and strengthened at the same time as you are reducing fat. But the application of exercise for weight management has other valuable benefits. Resistance training is particularly important to include for this reason. Increased muscle bulk also increases your resting metabolic rate, which helps reduce fat.

I am often asked if you can be fit but overweight. The answer is yes. If someone is overweight but physically fit, their risk of death is no greater than a person whose weight is in the normal range. You also get all of the other side benefits of regular exercise, including better mental health. That is not the case for someone who is in the healthy weight range but who is sedentary and unfit. However, even if you are fit, being overweight can have other health effects such as strain on your knee, hip and ankle joints.

OVEREXERCISING

A common misconception is that if a certain amount of exercise is good for you, then more is always better. Improving fitness relies on you pushing yourself beyond your usual physical load, because increasing the load results in bigger and faster biological changes.

There is a limit to the amount to which the body is able to adapt, however. Beyond this limit, your body does not have the chance to repair and recover. This is called 'overtraining'. While this is most likely to be seen in elite athletes, I also see it in keen amateurs who set their sights too high too soon, or people who become obsessed with training and do not have a well-planned training program that allows time for recovery.

If overtraining is a problem for you, it will create a counterproductive effect on your sense of wellbeing rather than the positive effect of a healthy level of exercise. It is about balance.

AVOIDING OVERTRAINING

- *get professional advice on your training program*
- *limit most exercise sessions to less than 60 minutes*
- *set aside one day each week as exercise free or very light recovery – walking, gentle aquafitness, tai chi*
- *mix up the types of exercise you do, so you avoid repeating the same program on consecutive days*
- *allow at least 48 hours between resistance training on the same muscle group*
- *measure your resting heart rate each morning on waking, to detect increases.*

HOW LONG WILL IT TAKE?

Let's assume you have the motivation to start exercising and you have found one activity or set of activities that you enjoy, or at least can learn to not hate. The next challenge is sustaining it. That often depends on you getting 'results'. So the question is: 'How long does it take to get results?'

This is a matter of what you are trying to achieve. If you simply want to feel happier, then every outing should have a small incremental effect.

Just the act of getting yourself up and going can be an achievement if you have been a chronic couch potato.

If weight loss is your aim, the goals of your exercise program will be intertwined with your nutritional plan. The amount of time it takes to reach your goal will depend on your starting weight, your target weight, and how long you take to get there. The aim would be to average half to one kilogram of weight loss per week.

If your aim is to feel physically fitter, expect to commit to a minimum 12-week process to see results in terms of stamina and strength. That is not to say you feel no different until the twelfth week, when you miraculously bounce out of bed and run a marathon. If you have been following the guidelines I set for you, over several weeks and months you will notice that the stairs are easier to climb, you are feeling more energetic during the day, you can lift loads you would not have been able to lift before and you will not feel breathless walking up a hill. It is important to try a range of different types of activity from walks to games of golf or tennis, dancing classes, yoga, bushwalking, surfing, swimming ... whatever takes your interest.

Think about your personality type. Are you the type of person who likes the solitude of walking alone with your thoughts or swimming laps of a pool? Or do you prefer to meet up with a group of bushwalkers? Are you happy with repeating one type of exercise each day or are you more the personality who likes to vary it so there is a different activity each day of the week?

Would a trainer or an exercise buddy help you to get out of bed in the morning to keep to a schedule? Do you have a physical disability that limits the type of exercise you are able to do?

If you are committed to achieving ultimate wellness, you will need to find a formula for daily activity that you enjoy, that gets you moving and that you are prepared to make a part of every day.

If you find you are skipping sessions or letting the routine go, carefully analyse the reason why that might be and think about how to overcome that obstacle.

Once you reach the 12-week mark, it is time to reassess your program to see if you have achieved your goals, and then set a new program with new goals or a sustainable maintenance plan that becomes your new normal routine.

MOVING FORWARD

Here are a few ideas from me for some goals you might like to set for yourself regarding exercise.

- *To exercise for 45 minutes to an hour every day using the plan in the exercise chapter*
- *To include weight/resistance training in my exercise program*
- *To include stretching in my exercise program*

YOUR GOALS

Goal	Activity	Obstacles/solutions	Result
To get fitter and lose 5 kg.	Start walking 45 minutes four times a week.	Finding time: arrange for partner to pick up kids on Tuesdays and Thursday. Go for a walk Saturday and Sunday.	After a month, not as breathless when I climb stairs. Fitness definitely improved! Have lost 2 kg.

IMMUNITY

As part of your Health Audit (page 15) you will need to consider how efficient your immune system is and what you can do to boost it. If your immune system is impaired, then you might be feeling tired and getting recurrent coughs and colds and other infections. An impaired immune system also increases the risk of developing a cancer.

Although it is tempting to think that you can just 'take something' to improve your health, boosting your immunity, like all other aspects of your health and wellbeing, is about a total approach to lifestyle rather than making a juice or taking a pill or going on a fad diet. Your immune system is incredibly complex and the state of your immunity depends on intricate interactions between your gut, your hormones, your respiratory tract, your other body systems and your emotional health.

There are two types of immunity: innate and adaptive.

Innate immunity involves your body's barriers to the outside world, including the skin and the lining of the gut and respiratory tract, as well as the body's responses to inflammation.

Adaptive immunity can take days or weeks to develop. This involves the production of antibodies or immunoglobulins in response to assault by potentially harmful invaders such as viruses or bacteria. The production of these antibodies allows for the future recognition of the same 'invaders' and a rapid response next time the immune system recognises them.

All of this activity requires certain raw materials to be available to the body, as well as efficiently functioning immune cells. Overactivity of your inflammatory response causes the immune system to wrongly recognise itself as foreign and mount a counterattack, resulting in autoimmune disease. Underactivity of your inflammatory response results in immune deficiency. If the immune system is underperforming, the result could be recurrent or unresolved infections, or the development of a cancer.

Immune cells of different types and the chemical messengers they respond to are able to turn the inflammatory response of the immune system up or down.

BOOSTING YOUR IMMUNITY

My advice, as always, is to check the fundamentals first. You might be surprised at how simple changes can give your immune system a lift.

✿ SLEEP

There is strong evidence that inadequate sleep is associated with a multitude of health problems, including mood disorders, cardiovascular disease and impaired immunity. The hormone melatonin is produced during sleep. Sleep disruption reduces the production of melatonin, which, with normal undisrupted sleep, in turn stimulates the production of a range of immune cells. Sleep deprivation activates your stress response.

✿ WEIGHT

Being underweight or overweight can impair your immune defences. We know that excess fat tissue is linked to low-grade systemic inflammation, type 2 diabetes and insulin resistance, heart disease, fatty liver disease and cancer.

✿ GUT

The state of your digestive system is critical to your immune responses. Your gut is the most important interface between your body and the external environment. It needs to make constant decisions about what is harmful, such as disease-causing bacteria, or harmless to you, such as food.

The lining of your gut is populated by billions of bacteria that constantly communicate with the cells in your immune system. So a healthy immune system depends on you having a healthy gut and a balance of beneficial bacteria.

✿ WATER

Every body process needs water. Make sure you drink about 1.5–2 litres a day. This might be in the form of water or teas.

✿ ALCOHOL

A small amount of alcohol, around one drink a day, may actually improve the immune system. But drinking excess alcohol leaches the body of nutrients important to the immune system, such as zinc.

Eat two serves of fruit and five serves of vegetables every day. Raw or lightly cooked is best. Dark colours, like berries and broccoli, tend to be higher in antioxidants. Eliminate junk foods that are high in calories and harmful ingredients, such as trans fats, but low in nutritional value.

Foods to include

Foods that enhance your immune function include fruit and vegetables; low GI foods; omega-3 rich foods such as fish; monounsaturated fats; nuts; green tea; small doses of alcohol; antioxidant-rich foods; herbs – garlic, ginger, cumin.

Foods to avoid

Foods that increase inflammation include excess kilojoules; high-GI foods; trans fats and saturated fats; salt; excessive alcohol; refined carbohydrates; dairy food; artificial colours, flavours and preservatives; gluten if you are gluten intolerant.

Spend some time in the outdoors

Vitamin D is an essential regulator of the immune system, yet it is one of the most common deficiencies I see. Vitamin D deficiency is strongly associated with an increased risk of 17 common cancers, autoimmune diseases (such as multiple sclerosis, type 1 diabetes, irritable bowel disease (IBD), rheumatoid arthritis), infectious diseases (tuberculosis), depression, hypertension, psoriasis and bone disorders (osteoporosis, osteomalacia and rickets). The simple antidote is regular time spent outdoors without overdoing the sun protection. That means sunshine without sunburn, for ideally 20 minutes a day on average.

Exercise without overexercising

Regular moderate aerobic and resistance activity enhance your immunity and reduce inflammation, whereas overtraining makes you more susceptible to infections and chronic fatigue.

Sort out stress

The immune system responds to the biochemical effects of emotions on your body. Excessive and unmanaged chronic stress leads to increased cortisol and suppressed immunity, increasing the likelihood of infections and cancer. Make sure you take time to look after yourself, spend time with friends who make you feel good about yourself and indulge in the things that bring you joy. Fix or eliminate toxic relationships. You may find you benefit from seeing a psychologist for help with managing your responses to stress.

Find time for stillness

Mindfulness meditation, yoga and tai chi are ways of helping this. Hypnosis, relaxation and guided imagery have been shown to be effective in cases of breast cancer, viral illnesses including chronic herpes simplex, and the common cold.

Environment

Check out your house for chemicals that you can eliminate from your environment. This might include household cleaning agents, paints and solvents, passive smoke, unnecessary pharmaceutical drugs – check with your doctor first – and plastic containers with Bisphenol A.

Investigate whether there are any sources of mould in your environment and take steps to remove it. Check around your workplace for sources of chemicals and see whether some can be changed to less toxic agents. (See 'Detox' section on page 51.)

HERBS AND SUPPLEMENTS

Many herbs and supplements help the body to improve immunity and resist disease.

The best way to correct nutritional deficiencies is by correcting dietary inadequacies with a balanced diet containing as much raw, whole and organic components as possible. Some people will need supplements to quickly correct significant deficiencies, such as iron or zinc. Vitamins A, B_6, B_{12}, C, D, E, folic acid and the trace elements iron, zinc, copper and selenium all work synergistically to support the protective activities of the immune cells. A multivitamin can assist with this. I recommend seeing a dietitian for an analysis of what you might be missing.

The mineral zinc is especially important for the healthy functioning of the immune system. Even mild zinc deficiency can result in impairment of your immune system.

Vitamin C has long been known to help immunity. Your body is not able to store vitamin C, so you need to eat or drink something containing vitamin C. If you exercise heavily, also take a supplement every day to maintain adequate levels.

Probiotics taken during pregnancy, infancy, when taking antibiotics and at times of illness will enhance your immunity by supporting the gut's role in your immune response. Different probiotics have different actions and so a variety of probiotics will need to be used depending on what you are trying to achieve.

There are many herbs known to enhance immunity. They include:

- *echinacea*
- *garlic*
- *astragalus*
- *andrographis* (Andrographis paniculata)
- *American ginseng* (Panax quinquefolius)
- *eleuthero* (Eleutherococcus senticosus)
- *green tea* (Camellia sinensis)

Professional advice is important in deciding doses, combinations and timing of taking herbs. Refer to the chapter 'Herbal Medicine', on page 233.

MOVING FORWARD

YOUR GOALS

Goal	Activity	Obstacle/solution	Result
Boost my immunity	Review the basics of my health	Finding the time to make the effort: fold these small things into my overall plan	I feel stronger and healthier

CONNECTION

Connectedness, spirituality and enriching your senses. On the surface, you might be wondering why I have included these subjects in a discussion of ultimate wellness. An integrative approach to your health and wellbeing would not be complete without paying attention to the connection between you and significant others, the connection of your senses to your environment, and a sense of faith about your connection to a greater philosophy of living.

SPIRITUALITY

'Spirituality' means different things to different people. You may take it to mean your philosophy of life, or the sum total of the things that matter to you and give your life meaning.

The framework for your spirituality may be in the form of a religion. But separate from religious spirituality might be the more secular descriptions of spirituality such as humanitarianism, love, compassion, tolerance, contentment or altruism.

Your brand of spirituality may express itself in your appreciation of nature, your pursuit of social justice, your relationships, your belief in a universal force or the study of science. It might be a combination of all the influences on your personal philosophy. However you express your spirituality, the things that give your life meaning, hope, comfort and peace of mind make up a very important element of emotional health and resilience.

Spiritual practices such as prayer, meditation, appreciation of nature and altruistic work increase your understanding of yourself and your place in the bigger picture. They also have a role to play in improving survival, coping and recovery. People with cancer who have a strong sense of spirituality have a more positive outlook, tend to be more satisfied with their lives and have greater ability to cope with pain.

Spirituality is one of those things that we often do not think about until we are faced with a life-threatening or life-challenging situation, such as the diagnosis of a serious illness. It is in these times that we are forced to dig deep to cope with adversity. How well we cope under these circumstances is a measure of our resilience.

So the question I will put to you is this: Why wait until a crisis to think about the place of spirituality in your life? Why not build your resilience by instilling important elements of spirituality into your life, to actually prepare you for adversity?

SPIRITUALITY AND WELLBEING

Some of the known health benefits of greater spirituality include:

- *reduced all-cause mortality and greater longevity*
- *reduced incidence of depression and quicker recovery from depressive episodes*
- *greater ability to cope with disability, illness and stress*
- *reduced substance abuse, including alcohol and illicit drugs, and modification of other risk factors, resulting in reductions in lifestyle-related illnesses*
- *reduced incidence of heart disease and hypertension*
- *reduced incidence of cancer and longer survival with cancer.*

SEEKING SPIRITUALITY

When it comes to lifting your health from 50 to 100, I can't just advise you to 'go and get spiritual'. What you can do is look at the things that you feel give your life meaning. This is not one of those things you can learn from a book – it requires self-reflection and raw honesty. You are the only person who can say what gives your life meaning; what really makes you happy or gives you an innate sense of peace.

I am often faced with a diagnostic challenge where someone tells me they feel depressed or anxious or exhausted, but my radar picks up an existential sadness rather than a medical diagnosis of depression or anxiety or chronic fatigue. Sure, you might feel sad or tired or nervous, but what lies beneath that? You are not going to get to the bottom of something like this in 10 or 15 minutes. Careful exploration is needed to discover what is missing that can cause such an 'absence of happiness'.

☘ LIFE GOALS

The Bucket List is a movie about two old men, played by Jack Nicholson and Morgan Freeman, who find out they have limited time left to live, and they set about doing all the things they ever wanted to do or dreamed of doing before they 'kicked the bucket'. The movie was the catalyst for a lot of people, including myself, to at least think about what was important in their lives, how they wanted to live the remainder of the time they had left, however short or long that time might be, and what they wanted to do before they died.

The really intriguing thing about that movie script is that although the pair travelled the world ticking off big-ticket items like jumping out of planes, flying over the North Pole, or visiting the Taj Mahal, in the end they discovered the more spiritually enriching things like 'helping a complete stranger for the good' and learning to appreciate the value of the love of their families were what gave them the greatest happiness.

You may think you are too young for a 'bucket list' of your own, but I think it is important at any age to develop a portfolio of dreams and goals. This can contain some of those 'big ticket' items like studying in Europe or driving around Australia. But chances are, if you think about it for a while, it will be the things that connect you to your 'significant others' in a more meaningful way, or that contribute something to the 'greater good' that will have the most spiritual meaning and ultimately do most for your emotional health.

A helpful exercise is to write a list of just five short-term goals, things you would like to experience or do or achieve in the next three months to a year.

Then think of another list of goals to cover a five-year timeframe.

Then write a list of five things you would like to achieve at some point in your life.

You can take your time coming up with these lists, and it should be an organic and evolving document that shifts with time. As you reach one goal, you can add another to replace it. If you reconsider your goals because your circumstances change, then the list may change from time to time until it develops into a truly meaningful plan for your future.

WHY BOTHER WITH SPIRITUALITY?

Medical research has turned its attention to the health effects of spirituality and has found that people who describe themselves as spiritual have a lower incidence of self-destructive behaviour like self-harming, suicide, smoking, drug and alcohol abuse and less stress-related illness. Spirituality has been shown to protect against depression and boost your immune system.

People undergoing heart surgery who consider themselves spiritual or religious are three times more likely to survive the surgery than people who do not have a spiritual framework.

ELEMENTS OF SPIRITUALITY

Improving your spiritual health is not about preventing or curing disease, it is about how you cope, regardless of your state of health. Searching for meaning or fulfilment is a very personal journey and has to be meaningful to you.

- *Think about what gives you positive feelings such as joy, comfort, hope, connectedness and strength.*
- *Develop a portfolio of achievable dreams and goals.*
- *Think about whether your work contributes in some positive way to others.*
- *Spend time in nature.*
- *Find time to 'do' some of the things that are important to you every day.*
- *Consider some altruistic work such as community volunteering.*
- *Have someone who will listen to your hopes, fears and dreams, and be there for others to express theirs.*
- *Think about the place of religion in your life and whether this might be incorporated in some way into your framework of spirituality.*
- *Reflect on whether faith – religion or spirituality – has been important in your past.*
- *Consider art and music appreciation in your daily life.*

CONNECTION WITH OTHERS

CONNECTEDNESS

Connectedness is literally about the connections you have with other people. Social connectedness is not always considered when we talk about the quality of your wellbeing, but it is an issue that has a really significant impact on your emotional and physical health.

You don't have to be a hermit in the bush and living off the land to lack human connections. My son works as a nurse in aged care and he tells me it breaks his heart to see some of the elderly people who are in their last months or years of life and rarely, if ever, get a visit from anyone other than the staff.

WHO ARE YOUR 3 AM PEOPLE?

There is a game we play with our children to get them thinking about connectedness. We ask the question: 'Who are our 3 am people?' Who are the people we could call in a crisis at 3 am without having to even think about whether they might get mad that we called and woke them from their sleep?

Your 3 am people might be family or friends. They will not be casual acquaintances. They might be people you see only occasionally, but you have a strong connection to them. For many people, biological family members would not appear on that list at all.

Your level of connectedness to the '3 am people' is how I would define your strongest connections. There is mutuality about the support you would give and expect from your closest people.

In medicine, we always ask patients for an emergency contact. I ask this question in addition to asking who the 'official' next of kin is, because they are often not the same person as the one you would contact any hour of the day or night if you had a medical emergency.

I have a friend who lives alone. She has family members, but she asked me if I would accept her medical Power of Attorney because she was not happy to give that responsibility to any of her family members who rarely see her and would not know what she would want to happen if she was desperately ill. I am one of her 3 am people, the people she would call in an emergency, not a family member.

CIRCLES OF CONNECTEDNESS

You could think about your connections like a series of circles inside circles. The people you place in each circle reflect the strength of your connection to them. You are the only person who can place the names in their appropriate circle. By appropriate, I mean the circle where *you* feel they belong, not the genetic likeness or where you think they would want to be, but where you *feel* those people are in relation to you.

The innermost circle is inhabited by your most intimate relationship. Ideally, this will be your partner. It may be a parent or an adult child, or it may your closest friend, or more than one of these.

Outside that circle is another circle with your 3 am friends. At this point, if you are counting on one hand you will almost certainly still have fingers left over.

Next are the friends and family you like spending time with but are a little more emotionally distant from you. You might call them at 7 am to tell them you have been taken to hospital.

Outside that group are the acquaintances you spend time with, but who do not share your personal information. They might find out about your crisis the next day from friends in the previous circle.

Beyond that are your work colleagues, contacts, hairdresser, shop-keepers, people you say hello to while you are walking the dog. There are the special purpose connections too, like support groups for specific health problems or social issues or the clubs you belong to.

In health care we are familiar with the power of connectedness in helping people manage in difficult times, or to recover from illness, with techniques such as support groups, group therapy and group education. Connectedness is about having a variety of these associations relevant to your stage of life and your social needs.

You can see the inherent need for social connectedness if you observe people in restaurants in the evenings. Eating in groups is a primitive instinct and you rarely see a single individual out to dinner in a restaurant. You might see a couple discussing the menu, ordering together, chatting while they wait for the food. Sometimes you will notice couples sitting through an entire meal and not speaking a word to each other, and not looking happy. Complete disconnect. There may be larger groups gathered to celebrate a birthday or a special event. We gather as groups to share happy occasions and to mourn. So you also see the need for connectedness at funerals. Friends and family gather to comfort each other in times of loss.

CONNECTING THROUGH SOCIAL MEDIA

In this era of communication technology, social networking sites like Facebook and Twitter, and texting and emails create the impression that people are more connected than ever before. But social networking by electronic means does not substitute for our need to connect with other people in person. Some of the loneliest people on the planet have loads of followers on Twitter and have 'friended' hundreds of people on Facebook.

While there's no substitute for actually seeing someone face to face, social media does allow people to reconnect and keep in touch who normally wouldn't stay in touch – for instance, old friends and families who are separated by distance. My youngest daughter asked me the other day what a 'pen-pal' was. It reminded me that we rarely pick up a pen to write to a friend, where just a few decades ago it was the common form of communication with friends or family living far away. Social media have also replaced the almost forgotten custom of writing letters.

People share interesting articles, jokes and news through Facebook and Twitter, and while it is not as good as sitting down and talking face to face, it does play an important role in being connected.

SOCIAL ISOLATION

The opposite of connectedness is social isolation or loneliness, which is closely linked with poor physical and mental health. Isolation is linked to increased risk of chronic disease, anxiety, depression, low productivity, substance abuse and domestic violence.

Loneliness is different from being alone. Sometimes we need time alone to pause, reflect, meditate, think and rest. In that 'alone' time we can still feel connected.

AUDIT YOUR CONNECTEDNESS

In the Health Audit, you answered some questions regarding the relationships in your life but a more detailed look can help. As an exercise on working out your level of connectedness and whether it might be impacting on how you are feeling, you can do a simple audit, which involves asking yourself some fundamental questions. Most of the questions are straightforward and uncomplicated, while others will need more reflection and perhaps be more challenging:

- *Do you have a primary relationship? How would you describe this relationship? See the questionnaire in the AUDIT section on page 15.*
- *Who lives at home with you?*
- *Describe your extended family.*
- *Have there been any stresses or difficulties with any of your relationships recently?*
- *In general, does contact with the important people in your life make you feel better or worse about yourself?*
- *What is your cultural/ethnic background and what effect does this have on your life?*

- *How do you contact people who are important to you and how much time do you spend each week interacting with them?*
- *Who are your 3 am people?*
- *Who do you trust to talk to about your concerns or problems?*
- *Do the people you spend time with make you feel valued and loved?*
- *Describe your workplace and the interactions with colleagues. Are there any conflicts or stresses with the people there?*
- *Do you love your job and do you look forward to going to work each day?*
- *How closely do you identify with your place of work? Is it 'just a job' or is it something you feel proud to be associated with?*
- *What social activities do you have and how often?*
- *What non-work-related interests and hobbies do you have?*
- *What memberships do you have to clubs or organisations? What time do you spend there and what sort of activities do you do?*
- *What is your financial situation?*
- *What part, if any, does religion or spirituality play in your life?*

You don't need to 'tick all the boxes', but thinking about all of these aspects of connectedness will give you an idea of the breadth of connections you have and the impact they have on your life. Hopefully the exercise will get you thinking about some of the areas you can plan to address.

Once you have conducted the audit of your own connectedness, you will have some clues about what to do to improve your sense of connectedness. The following recommendations are some of the ways you can address problems with connectedness.

❧ FIND YOUR TRIBE

Consider the collective noun 'tribe'. It is no coincidence that there are so many distinct names to describe a collection of a particular species: a pod of dolphins, a school of fish, a pride of lions, a parliament of owls. When I am kayaking I have the chance to observe natural connections, the way species of the same type cluster together and behave independently but collectively.

We all need to find our collective noun.

Has there ever been a time in your life when you have looked around you and thought, 'What am I doing here? I don't belong here.' I know I have.

You are faced with two choices: stay and adapt your outside appearance but know in your heart that you don't belong; or go and find your tribe.

By this I mean look around at different groups or clusters of people who share a common interest, or a philosophy, or a way of living that feels like a good fit for you. Defining a sense of belonging is hard, but your connectedness can be increased by finding the tribe that makes you feel like you automatically belong. This might be your family of origin, but it might also be the group of people you gather around yourself.

I have met many young gay people who felt socially isolated in their families and communities because they felt 'different': not belonging in their environment at home or at school, unable to express themselves or feeling the fear of rejection, or having been subject to bullying. Some become depressed, some attempt suicide. Many leave their home towns in search of a social environment where they can feel accepted and 'connected'.

Another common phenomenon is the loneliness and social isolation of elderly people who become widowed, who outlive the friendships of their younger years and who may have lost the connections with their cultural origins. Elderly people find it more difficult to make new friendships or establish new networks. This results in a gradual loss of connectedness and development of loneliness and depression.

☘ MEND OR END DAMAGING RELATIONSHIPS

Some of the loneliest people I have met are in unhappy or unfulfilling relationships – not bad enough to leave but not good enough to stay – or are 'living their own lives'. Research has shown us that living in an unhappy relationship is a significant risk factor for death – yes, death – from a whole range of different causes.

On the other hand, we know that happy and stable relationships result in better functioning of the immune system. Social support in the form of marriage or a committed long-term relationship, or frequent daily contact with other people, plus the presence of a close confidant, have been demonstrated to have a protective effect against the progression of cancer. The real issue here is not the quantity of relationships and connections, but their quality.

A recent meta-analysis looked at the extent to which social relationships influence the risk for mortality and found a 50 per cent increased likelihood of survival in people with stronger social relationships, an effect that is comparable with the more recognised 'lifestyle' risk factors such as smoking or alcohol consumption.

❦ ELIMINATE HOSTILITY

Think about sources of conflict or hostility in your life. Think about the last time you had an argument with a significant person in your life, perhaps your mother? Was it over something minor? Did it escalate into a screaming match, with angry emails fired back and forth and other family members recruited to take sides?

What about holiday times? Do you look forward to going back home for Christmas or weddings or other family celebrations, or do you dread it? If you dread the prospect of visiting your family of origin, then it will be affecting your general wellbeing.

If there is a person in your inner circles who causes you angst a lot of the time, then you need to work out why that is happening, whether it can be avoided, or whether the underlying problem can be fixed. This may need professional guidance from a trained counsellor.

When relationships are damaging to your wellbeing, the worst thing you can do is to do nothing, to just let things go on upsetting you. With the help of advice from a close friend or a counsellor, mend the relationship problems or end the relationship and move on.

Hostility in relationships can range in severity from simple disagreements through persistent aggravation and, finally, to all-out war. The ultimate failure of conflict resolution is war. War does not exclusively mean overt acts of aggression between nations: on a metaphorical level, war can be an unresolved conflict between two people, two conflicting ideologies, or even within an individual. If the underlying source of conflict cannot be resolved, then retreat can be a noble form of victory and a way of protecting yourself. So, mend it or end it.

❦ FORGIVE

Forgiveness is a term that seems to have a place more in religious texts than in health and wellbeing advice, but when it comes to connectedness and emotional health, it is a concept worth exploring. I have mentioned the importance of moving on from damaging and irreparable relationships.

An essential prerequisite for moving on is to let go of resentment, bitterness, anger or plans for retribution. These negative emotions will eat at your emotional and physical wellbeing, and contribute to high blood pressure, anxiety, depression, insomnia and alcohol and other substance abuse.

Ending a grudge can be difficult if the person who caused you hurt does not accept responsibility for the effect of their behaviour or refuses to see your point of view. In fact, holding a grudge gives all the power to the person who hurt you.

It is important to know that forgiveness does not always involve reconciliation. In fact, it might require distancing so that you can focus on how you are feeling, rather than trying to force the other person to see things from your perspective.

The specific techniques for forgiveness are more complicated than saying, 'Just move on.' You may need professional guidance to be able to put your grievances in perspective in a way that is healthy for you so that you can move on. Once you do let go of that negativity, you can take more control of your emotional life and make space for positive aspects of life, such as kindness, compassion, optimism and peace.

For your own sake, forgive past grievances, whether they can be resolved or not. See the chapter on Stress and mental health on page 90 for more details about counselling.

❧ REACH OUT

I remember when I was a young mother. I was in the first year out of medical school and all my university friends and professional contacts were, at that stage, childless and getting on with their careers. I had moved to a part of Sydney that was away from my family and old friends. Nobody I knew had babies.

It was a confusing and lonely time. In retrospect, I recognise that I felt quite depressed. I still remember how hard it was to pick up the phone and call the number for the local parents' group. I resisted having to make new friends because I was going back to work in six months, but I felt so isolated. I was acutely aware of the need for a touchstone, for other people around my age who were going through similar experiences.

The first group I tried out just wasn't on my wavelength. We had nothing in common except we all had babies. The second group was the same. I almost gave up but a friend of a friend suggested I try a group a few suburbs away. The pieces fell into place. I met some other young professional women with babies who were taking time off work before returning to their careers. That connection made all the difference to my experience of early parenting and resulted in some long-term friendships.

Reaching out and making connections with other people is easier for some personality types than others. Plus it gets more difficult to establish new friendships and social networks as you get older. If you want to feel the best you can, even if it is difficult for you, you are going to need to work out a way of reaching out.

In my clinical practice, I see quite a few expats, business people and their families who are transferred from one country to another every few years for their work. These expats are very practised at finding a tribe and quickly establishing new connections. You don't have to move cities or countries to establish new and meaningful connections. I also see many retired and elderly people who are engaged in all sorts of activities and volunteer community work.

Where to go to make new connections:

- **Work.** *Look around your workplace and see if there are people you would like to get to know better. Go along to social events such as after-work drinks.*

- **Sport.** *Think of a sport or activity you enjoyed in the past, or an activity you might like to learn, like golf or lawn bowls or dancing classes. Sports clubs can be a great way to meet people with a shared interest. Exchange contact details with people you meet so that you can arrange a game in your free time.*

- **Volunteer.** *Charities and community groups rely on the time donated by members of the community to provide their services. Look for a cause or charity that has meaning for you and sign up.*

- **Altruism and other acts of kindness.** *Reaching out to others without the expectation of anything in return not only makes you feel good, it increases what we call 'social capital' – a contribution or gift to benefit your community – and brings with it the possibility of meaningful connectedness.*

- **Use your existing network.** *Your network of contacts can introduce you to new people outside your usual routines.*

- **Turn up.** *If you are invited to a social event, make the effort to go, even if you don't feel like it.*

❧ MAKING NEW FRIENDS

- **Do not expect instant friendships.** *Good friends don't happen overnight. Start with a conversation about your interests.*
- **Do not disclose deeply personal issues too soon.** *Wait until you know the other person and their trustworthiness before you share your deeper thoughts and feelings.*
- **Accept differences.** *Recognise that other people might have different attitudes and experiences, and see them as providing texture to your own life and experiences.*
- **Stay true to your core beliefs.** *Avoid sacrificing your core beliefs or morals in an effort to fit in with a new group.*
- **Avoid gossip.** *If a new friend divulges a personal matter, respect their confidentiality.*

❧ KEEPING FRIENDS

Sometimes we forget to nurture the established friendships we made in the past. Reaching out can also mean reaching back into past friendships where you may have lost contact through following different paths in life, or just 'getting busy'. This means taking the time to check up on your friends, see what they are up to, listen to their problems and offer support. Show interest in their lives. Social media can help you to reconnect.

❧ YOUR HOME LIFE

If you are living alone and feeling lonely, consider home-sharing or multi-generational housing options. This is not just for young people.

Once you have completed your personal connectedness audit, think about the quantity and quality of your connections with other people. If you believe there is room for improvement, and there almost always is, then you have found another area of your life in which to achieve your ultimate level of wellbeing.

CONNECTION WITH SENSES

COME TO YOUR SENSES

A few years ago I was at a function for the Australian Medical Association and one of my colleagues there, an ophthalmologist, was telling me about an elderly patient he had been asked to see in a nursing home. This woman had not communicated with anyone for many, many months. She never spoke or smiled. She did not interact with staff, other residents or even her family. She sat in a corner from the time she was helped out of bed until she went back to bed at night. It was thought she had developed dementia.

A specialist eye surgeon, my friend was asked to ascertain whether there was any possibility that her vision was contributing to her behaviour because she was known to have cataracts and hearing impairment. The idea was that if her sight could be restored just enough to see the television, even if reading a book was beyond her, then it would help her pass her time. He examined her and confirmed the cataracts, and agreed to do the operation, despite the fact it would be difficult to know how the retina would function once the cataract was removed.

The surgery went without a hitch. When he unfurled the bandage and peeled back the eye patch, the question was answered. The widest and most beautiful, joyous smile lit up the patient's face as she caught sight of her daughter and grandchildren for the first time in many years.

Trapped in a prison of progressive blindness and profound deafness for years had rendered her unable to communicate with her surroundings. Removing the cataract from one of her eyes let in the light and enabled her to see the faces of her children and grandchildren, to be entertained by television and to read again.

The official term for this condition is 'sensory deprivation'. It is also described as 'perceptual isolation'. Literally, it means depriving the senses of stimulation.

The extreme case of sensory deprivation is the elimination or drastic reduction in sensory input. Subjection to this for long enough can result in extreme anxiety, depression, apathy, hallucinations and bizarre thinking patterns.

FIVE SENSES

Our senses are the input channels for our perception and understanding of our environment. They are our interface with the rest of the world. The reason I tell you this is to remind you that we have five senses, and that if any one of them is underperforming or out of action, it is important to do whatever you can to reinvigorate it or compensate for it in some way by enhancing the stimulation and functioning of the remaining senses.

It is not just the quantity of stimulation that can have an effect on your wellbeing, but also the quality of that sensory input. We tend to fall into a rut of doing the same things and going through the same routines without variation, or failing to concentrate on the most fundamental of needs, such as human touch.

Try this exercise. Make a list of your five senses. Over the course of the day, note down the things you do to enhance or stimulate any of them. Once you have done that, think of ways you can vary or enrich your sensory experiences.

SIGHT

The true story I told you about the elderly woman in the nursing home who, deprived of sensory input from her eyes and ears became socially isolated and withdrawn, is an example of the consequences of the loss of one or more of your senses. Blindness is at the extreme end of the spectrum of visual loss.

As we age, our vision can become less acute and it can be more difficult to see a sharp image. Lots of things can go wrong with the eyes to contribute to this failing visual acuity, so regular vision testing is important to stay on top of any problems and make sure they are monitored and treated. Protecting your eyesight is an essential investment in your future wellbeing.

The question, then, is how to make the most of this important sense. Sure, you use your eyes to get around, read and watch television, but think about what else you can do to enrich your visual inputs. Look at the colours in your home and think about the feelings those colours evoke. Do you like the colours of the paintwork, furniture, fabrics, ornaments and accessories? Is your home neat and tidy or does it look chaotic?

Many of us have routines that keep us spending most of the day indoors in rigid, unchanging built environments. The richest source of visual input

Protecting your eyesight

- Wear eye protection for work and sport to avoid injury.
- Don't smoke.
- Arrange regular eye checks, particularly for glaucoma and cataract.
- Maintain healthy blood glucose levels. Diabetes affects vision.
- Wear sun-protective sunglasses, especially if you spend a lot of time outdoors.
- Eat a low-fat diet – elevated cholesterol is a risk factor for macular degeneration and complications of diabetes.
- Eat a diet high in lutein and zeaxanthin – carotenoids that give plants their orange, red or yellow colour – fish and green leafy vegetables.
- Eat high intakes of omega-3 polyunsaturated fatty acids to reduce the risk of cataract.
- Adequate dietary protein may reduce the risk of one form of cataract.

is nature. The complex geometry of nature provides the richest source of visual stimulation with its infinite array of shapes and colours, stimulating the entire visual field rather than a small area of focus.

Make exposing yourself to visual stimuli from nature an important part of every day. Depending on where you live, go for a walk, a swim or surf, or just sit quietly in a place where you can see trees and the sky some time during the day to improve your sense of wellbeing.

☘ HEARING

For those of us born with normal hearing, hearing loss does not have to be inevitable as we age, although it does tend to become more likely. Hearing loss can be so gradual you hardly notice it, until you realise you are asking people to repeat what they are saying and you find it difficult to follow conversations in a noisy restaurant or a crowd. Or maybe you are told you have the television volume turned up very loud.

When I raise the issue of hearing in my practice, I commonly find that family members have been trying to get the patient to have their hearing tested or try a hearing aid for ages. Their efforts have been met with a flat denial or fierce resistance to there being a hearing problem, or that the patient would never consider a hearing aid because 'That's for old people'.

It is common to hear about frustration and outright anger caused by a member of a relationship or family refusing to address the problem their hearing loss is creating not just for themselves but for other people trying

Causes of hearing loss

- **Blocked ear canal.** The ear canal can be blocked by ear wax, infection, or bony growths called exostoses. Hearing will be reduced in one or both ears. There may be a sense of fullness in the ear, tinnitus or ringing in the ears, and feeling off balance. If infection is present, there may be pain.
- **Noise-induced deafness.** Common sources of noise exposure are loud music – concerts and MP3 players – industrial machinery, and military or other weapons. Sometimes there is temporary hearing loss after exposure to loud noise. Onset of tinnitus is commonly associated. The hearing loss becomes permanent if there is continued exposure.
- **Middle ear infection.** Infection can travel from the back of the throat up the Eustachian tube to the middle ear. Hearing loss in children can affect speech development. Earache usually follows or is associated with a respiratory infection and a fever, with loss of hearing that comes on at the time of the infection. Hearing loss may become chronic.
- **Ageing, or presbyacusis.** By age 65, approximately 31 per cent of the population has significant age-related hearing loss, increasing to 50 per cent by age 75. Exhibited by gradual progressive difficulty hearing speech in an older person, especially in noisy environments. The problem starts with higher frequency sounds. The TV or music is up too loud for others and social withdrawal is common.
- **Drug side effect.** Drugs known to cause deafness include antibiotics, such as gentamicin and tobramycin, diuretics (frusemide), chemotherapy, quinine and aspirin. Hearing loss comes on after starting a medication known to cause toxicity to the ear.

to communicate with them on a daily basis. One man whose family had been trying to encourage him to have his hearing checked told me that the movie he had enjoyed most in years was *The Artist* (2012), the French silent movie. That was because he did not have to strain to hear and there wasn't any dialogue to follow.

Losing your hearing acuity can have a gradual damaging effect on your quality of life and your relationships. Problems such as social isolation, depression, anxiety, loneliness and stress within relationships are closely linked with hearing loss.

Protecting your hearing

Avoid injuring the ear canal with cotton buds. If you produce a lot of wax, you may need to use a wax softening drop regularly, once or twice a week.

- *Reduce exposure to environmental noise by avoiding loud music, wearing earplugs – special earplugs are available that allow appreciation of music but reduce noise reaching the ear – or headphones in noisy environments and occupations. Limit the volume on MP3 players. This is particularly important in young children.*

- *Avoid exposure to tobacco smoke.*

- *Avoid close contact with people with respiratory infections.*

- *Ensure good nutrition.*

- *Maintain healthy lifestyle habits, including eating a healthy low-fat diet. Treat any chronic medical conditions, like high blood pressure or diabetes.*

- *Avoid medications known to cause hearing loss unless there is no other option and benefit outweighs the risk. This is particularly important if you have an existing hearing problem.*

It is important to think about periods of stillness and the appropriate auditory stimulation to create the ambience you want at home and at work. Working out what effect different types of sound input have on your emotions, and the mood you want to create at a particular time according to your preferences, may take a little planning.

Auditory stimulation might involve conversation, classical music or different styles of popular music. Some people love the sound of children playing but others find it irritating. The chirping of birds in the trees or the sound of gently lapping waves can be very calming.

In this time of mobile personal sound devices, where almost everyone walks around with earbud headphones or where for urban dwellers there is loud traffic noise and crowds, it is equally important to find periods of stillness and peace with minimal or very gentle auditory input.

❧ TOUCH

Tactile stimulation is important to wellbeing at every age, from birth to the process of dying. If you were deprived of touch as a child, you are more likely as an adult to be depressed, anxious, angry and aggressive. Deprived of touch as an adult, you can become depressed and anxious.

The highest risk of touch deprivation is in the elderly, in particular those people who are widowed, or separated by disability and confined to a residential aged-care facility. They might have someone to wash and dress them, but the caring touch is often lacking: holding a hand, having a hug, stroking an arm. Healing touch has been recognised in religious texts as 'the laying on of hands'. Without it, you see a condition called 'skin hunger', and emotional response to the unmet need for physical contact. This is quite distinct from sexual need.

If you are in a relationship, you may be having sex but craving intimacy and affection. Spending more time simply touching or hugging has a powerful effect on relaxing and reducing stress.

The sensation of touch is different from the form of therapy known as 'therapeutic touch', a so-called energy therapy sometimes recommended for treatment of pain and anxiety but which has yet to be comprehensively studied for effectiveness. Therapeutic massage uses a form of touch to relax muscles and relieve pain, rehabilitate from injury and reduce stress.

If you are going to try massage, make sure the massage therapist is appropriately trained. If you have any doubt about whether massage is appropriate for you, ask your doctor.

❧ TASTE

Eating is about much more than just getting enough of the right food into you to give you energy and keep you well, it is also about taste, which is the ability to detect flavours through the sensory organs on your tongue called tastebuds. Taste is traditionally divided into five components: sweet, sour, bitter, salty and savoury. It is also affected by the texture and temperature of food and drinks.

We tend to take the sensation of taste for granted until it is gone. Actually, some patients I see don't realise their sense of taste has gone until we test it. This is because an intact sense of smell often compensates for a reduced sense of taste.

A low zinc level can affect the sense of taste, and once we restore zinc levels in people who have been deficient, they notice their taste returns. Perhaps the most reliable measure of zinc levels in the body is to swish a solution of zinc around in your mouth. If you have adequate zinc levels, you will notice an immediate strong taste. If you have a deficiency, the solution will taste like water.

Other medical conditions that can affect taste sensation include niacin deficiency, multiple sclerosis and other neurological conditions, diabetes and hypothyroidism. Cigarette smoking and inflammation of the tongue can affect taste too. The possibility of a drug side effect can also be a contributing cause.

Interestingly, people who lose their sense of taste find their appetite is decreased, so taste has a lot to do with maintaining healthy nutrition.

But what about if you have a normal sense of taste? What can you do to stimulate that sense?

Try doing an audit of all the things you eat, drink and put into your mouth for about three days to see if there is a narrow or a wide variety of tastes. Check your pantry and refrigerator. Do you have a broad range of different tastes and a good-sized collection of herbs and spices to add to your food? Look at some recipe books to see what spices you could add to the meals you prepare and pick them up on your next trip to the supermarket. Also try to branch out with more variety in the foods you buy or the meals you order to stimulate your taste.

🌿 SMELL

Different smells have different meaning for different people, and they can evoke powerful emotions and memories. They can also create physiological effects. Subtle effects on 'feeling' are very qualitative and impossible to accurately measure.

Real estate agents know the power of aromatherapy in creating an ambience for selling a house. The aroma of freshly roasted coffee, or bread baking in the oven, fresh flowers or essential oils in a house can create a strong sensory impression and reactions in potential buyers.

Essential oils can be added to massage oils, dropped into bathwater, or heated in water to diffuse into the atmosphere. As one example, lavender has long been used for sleep disorders and anxiety. Studies have shown that lavender aromatherapy induces a state of relaxation in healthy people, and reduces agitation in the elderly with dementia.

When you have a massage with essential oils, the massage therapist may ask you to choose from a range of aromas based on your preference. Your choice will depend on how the aroma makes you feel, emotionally and physically.

Think about the smells that make you feel happy, calm or relaxed. Then consider how you might be able to include those aromas in your home or workplace to stimulate your sense of smell.

❧ SIXTH SENSE

At the risk of sounding 'new age-y', I would like you to pause for a moment to reflect on the importance of your so-called 'sixth sense'. Another name for this might be intuition.

I suppose I could describe myself as an 'intuitive diagnostician'. Obviously, intuition gets better with time and improves with experience, but I make sure I pay careful attention to my initial impressions of whether there is a serious problem with a patient and what might be going on. It is based on things like a patient's demeanour, their facial expressions, the way they get up from the chair in the waiting room, how they walk, the way they speak, how they breathe, the subtleties of body language.

Similarly, I listen to what patients tell me about their 'feeling' that something is wrong. Then we have to work out what that might be. I have had women ask me for a breast check and a mammogram, even though they are not at 'recommended screening age', because they have a feeling there is something wrong – no pain, no lump to find, just a sense there is a problem – and found a breast cancer.

Much of intuition is a response to an elaborate combination of subconscious cues informed by experience. This is a principle you can take on board. If you tap into your 'sixth sense', trust your instincts and take action, you can find the way to improve your wellbeing and happiness.

OTHER SENSES

I want you to think about another five senses we might enrich. They are wisely called 'senses' because they inform and influence the ways we communicate with the world and the people around us. Thinking about these other senses may give you more ideas about how you can increase your happiness and general wellbeing.

❧ SENSE OF ADVENTURE

How about the sense of adventure? As we grow older, we tend to become more risk averse. On the one hand, it is a sign of maturity born of experience to be more aware of physical, emotional and financial risk. But you don't have to want to go mushing with huskies in the Arctic or dangling off a nauseatingly high cliff or jumping out of planes to have a sense of adventure. The other way to look at it is that life presents us with unlimited opportunities for adventures with little downside.

Adventure can be about widening your sphere of experiences of the world, trying new and unfamiliar things, and thinking of activities outside your usual routines. A defined area of the brain is activated when we choose unfamiliar options. Facing something you fear and summoning the courage to do that thing can help you to discover your potential and improve your ability to make complex decisions in an uncertain situation.

❧ SENSE OF HUMOUR

They say laughter is the best medicine, and a sense of humour is the ability to provoke laughter in others or see amusement in unexpected or quirky situations. Maintaining a sense of humour through difficult times helps to reduce your stress levels.

Laughter has positive health benefits. It reduces stress hormone levels, enhances creativity, improves mood, increases pain tolerance, reduces blood pressure and improves immune function.

The Australian government felt the need to define the Australian sense of humour as an element of the Australian character on its website. Yes, there is a page on the government's website devoted to the Australian sense of humour. It is said to be 'dry, full of extremes, anti-authoritarian, self-mocking and ironic'.

Interestingly, putting aside individual perception, there are strong cultural and geographic differences in what we find funny. What cultures have in common is probably the more important factor, and that is the effect of laughter on connectedness.

❧ SENSE OF WONDER

Technically speaking, a sense of wonder can be defined as a feeling of awakening or awe triggered by an expansion of your awareness of what is possible. As we get older and gather experience, it is not possible to go back to a state of naivety and experience the 'old' again as 'new', so it takes more to impress us. But it is possible to experience a sense of wonder in our everyday lives amongst all our responsibilities and routines.

If you want to rediscover your sense of wonder, spend time with a child and see the world through their eyes. Or take on a creative pursuit. The process of creating art, music, poetry or prose might just surprise you.

Travel is an obvious way to step outside the expected and marvel at natural landscapes and alternative cultures. But you don't need to travel far to experience wonder. Sometimes just stopping to look at a rainbow, or a cloud formation, or a sunset can be a source of awe.

❧ SENSE OF ACHIEVEMENT

Achievement is the result of preparation, hard work and opportunity. Knowing where you are going helps, so it is important to set yourself realistic goals with reasonable timeframes. In the pursuit of ever-greater goals, take pause every so often to appreciate what you have achieved.

The sources of your sense of achievement are deeply personal. I remember a conversation with a woman who had been feeling that she had achieved little. Several of her friends were high-powered professional women and many women she knew had at least one university degree. She had made the choice to be a wife and mother, a role she felt she carried out to the best of her ability. Reflecting on the results of her work, her four children, a happy marriage and a well-run home, she was able to feel a sense of achievement for having done her job to the best of her ability and having met her goals.

For those of us who are professionally ambitious, it is important to stop to reflect every so often on the goals you have achieved, even as you envisage the next one.

Expressing a sense of gratitude for all that is good and right in your life is a time-honoured tradition in every culture and religion. Saying grace, the American tradition of Thanksgiving, the Jewish Berakhot, and a multitude of other customs enable us to express our thanks for blessings or good fortune or for the provision of life's basics.

It can be easy to become jaded and dissatisfied with life. Instead, find a balance between the things you still want to achieve or attain, and being thankful for the things you have. Think of it as stopping to reflect on what I call the 'donut rather than the hole'. This may be framed as a religious rite or a personal reflection. Gratitude can also be expressed in a written note or a phone call thanking someone for a favour, a kindness or a gift.

However it is expressed, genuine gratitude increases happiness and helps to build bonds of friendship. A conscious effort to express and feel gratitude can also combat feelings of negativity, anger and resentment.

So come to your senses, and enjoy the benefits of feeling so much better.

MOVING FORWARD

Here are a few suggestions from me for some goals you might like to set yourself regarding connectedness.

- *To consider the role of spirituality within my own life*
- *To reinforce connections with my friends, family, colleagues and community*
- *To join a club or interest group or professional association*
- *To make a plan for enriching every one of my senses every day. Not just the five senses of touch, hearing, sight, smell and taste … but all those other senses that can fall by the wayside of a busy life … sense of humour, sense of adventure, sense of wonder.*
- *Very soon, I hope you can add 'sense of achievement' by fulfilling my ultimate wellness goals.*

YOUR GOALS

Goal	Activity	Obstacles/Solutions	Result
To increase my sense of connection	Renew old friendships. Make an effort to make new ones.	It's harder when you are older to make new friends: join a sporting club.	I feel happier in my self and my life.

Integrative medicine and complementary treatments

Integrative medicine is a philosophy of health care that takes the broadest possible view of the causes of health and disease, has a focus on prevention and incorporates the best available evidence-based forms of treatment. It takes into account patients' experiences and preferences. In this section I will discuss with you how you can use integrative medicine and complementary treatments to enhance your health in a sensible, safe and informed manner.

ACUPUNCTURE AND PHYSICAL THERAPIES

COULD ACUPUNCTURE BE RIGHT FOR ME?

The conditions for which I most commonly recommend acupuncture are:

- *back and neck pain*
- *assisting fertility*
- *menopausal hot flushes not responding to herbal medicines*
- *chronic pain*
- *pregnancy-related nausea*
- *managing nausea from chemotherapy*
- *musculoskeletal problems and headaches.*

These are not the only conditions where acupuncture can be useful and you need to discuss with your doctor or acupuncturist whether it might help you. The big advantage is that when it works for you, acupuncture can reduce or eliminate the need for medication. This is particularly important in conditions like pregnancy, insomnia and musculoskeletal pain.

There was a time not so long ago when acupuncture was viewed by my medical colleagues as a bit of a 'dark art' and treated with suspicion and scepticism. How could sticking a few little needles in seemingly random parts of someone's body block pain, relieve symptoms or cure illness? How could it have any more action than a placebo effect? The sceptics are still out there trying to dampen enthusiasm for this ancient Traditional Chinese Medicine (TCM) technique, but its popularity speaks volumes and scientific evidence is growing.

Just as an aside, a few years ago one of my toy poodles, Lulu, was very sick. She had had a severe gut problem and, despite standard veterinary treatment, after several months she was still having problems with abdominal pain. So we took her to a veterinary acupuncturist. Within seconds of the acupuncture needles being inserted, she completely relaxed and fell asleep. Whether it was the acupuncture, or the Chinese herbs the vet supplied, or the combination of the two that made her better, I am not sure, but she turned the corner quickly and was back to her normal self soon after those treatments.

It is important to place acupuncture within the full range of TCM practices developed over thousands of years, and to have a basic understanding of its underlying theory.

How or why acupuncture works is difficult to explain because it is based on the TCM concept if qi – pronounced 'chee' – or energy in the body that is conducted along pathways or meridians, between the surface of the body and the internal organs. The meridians are not anatomical points as we understand them in Western medicine.

Acupuncture points are positions on the skin all over the body that correspond to these meridians. All TCM practices, including acupuncture, aim to strengthen the flow of qi. One of the difficulties in finding a medical explanation for acupuncture is that the system of meridians does not correspond at all to the physiological structure or language of Western medicine.

TCM uses eight principles to assess symptoms and categorise conditions: cold/heat; interior/exterior; excess/deficiency; and yin/yang, the chief principles. A TCM consultation will usually begin with a history of your health problem and then your pulse is taken on both arms and your tongue is inspected. The qualities of the pulse gives the practitioner a guide to what might be going wrong. Then thin, flexible needles are inserted in selected positions on your body.

Acupuncture aims to re-establish a balance between two opposing but complementary forces in all life forms and in the environment, and to encourage the body to heal itself – the 'Yin-Yang' theory. TCM also uses the five elements theory – fire, earth, metal, water and wood – to explain how the body works; these elements correspond to particular organs and tissues in the body.

Other TCM therapies used by a TCM practitioner in conjunction with acupuncture include moxibustion, burning moxa – a cone or stick of dried herb, usually mugwort – on or near the skin, sometimes in conjunction with acupuncture; cupping, applying a heated cup to the skin to create a slight suction; Chinese massage; mind–body therapies such as qi gong and tai chi; and dietary therapy.

These days there are a lot of doctors and physiotherapists who have taken postgraduate training in acupuncture and offer it as a part of their treatment protocols. It has become such a common treatment in Western medicine now that many former sceptics are saying that it could be considered mainstream medicine.

It is not enough to say 'acupuncture works'. We need to be far more specific and say what acupuncture works *for*, and where it is probably not effective, or not as effective as other treatments. What medical science has been able to add to centuries of experience is a refinement of where acupuncture is likely to be most effective.

Standard scientific studies are difficult but not impossible because of the challenge of providing what we call a 'placebo control'. For many conditions where acupuncture can be used, the evidence has not been systematically reviewed, or the current scientific evidence to prove that it is effective is not yet established.

The National Institutes of Health in the United States released a consensus statement on the evidence for the use of acupuncture to treat or manage a range of disorders. They found that there was evidence that acupuncture is effective to treat post-operative and chemotherapy nausea and vomiting, nausea of pregnancy, and post-operative dental pain. The panel also concluded in their consensus statement that there are a number of other pain-related conditions for which acupuncture may be effective as an adjunct therapy, an acceptable alternative, or as part of a comprehensive treatment program, but for which there is less convincing scientific data. These conditions include but are not limited to:

- *addiction*
- *stroke rehabilitation*
- *headache*
- *menstrual cramps*
- *tennis elbow*
- *fibromyalgia or general muscle pain*
- *lower back pain*
- *carpal tunnel syndrome*
- *asthma.*

Even if you think you would hate acupuncture because you are afraid of needles, it can be worthwhile giving it a try. I was reluctant at first myself, but it really is virtually painless because the needles are so fine. Occasionally the practitioner will strike a spot that hurts but it quickly settles down or they move the needle.

Not all acupuncturists are doctors and not all doctors practise acupuncture. From July 2012, TCM practitioners have been registered nationally as a profession in Australia. That does not guarantee that a practitioner will have had a comprehensive university education, because some practitioners have been 'grandfathered' onto the register as they have been working as TCM practitioners for many years.

To make sure the practitioner you are seeing has a minimum level of qualification, check that they have graduated from a reputable university and that they are registered with their appropriate professional body to practise acupuncture. These days it should go without saying, but ensure that the practitioner uses new disposable needles discarded after each treatment.

Let your acupuncturist know if you are pregnant, or likely to be pregnant. And make sure you tell your doctor and other health practitioners if you are using TCM, and let your TCM practitioner know of your medical therapies.

OTHER PHYSICAL THERAPIES

Throughout the process of reading this book and auditing your health, you will have been carefully considering your current health status and your health goals. Physical therapies may help you to solve particular health problems and achieve your health goals.

When people ask me about which physical therapy might be best for them, sometimes it can be difficult to give them a simple answer. You might be thinking about physical therapy for the relief of musculoskeletal injuries, aches and pains, stiffness or weakness. Or it might be as part of your recovery from injury or surgery.

If you find it difficult to choose between the different types of physical therapies in deciding what to do, then that is perfectly understandable. There is a lot of crossover between them. While each therapy is a separate discipline with its own history and philosophy, they all borrow techniques from each other as they evolve, so they have a lot of common features.

If you have a musculoskeletal problem or injury, you can see a physical therapist directly. If you are not sure of the nature of the problem, or do not know who would best suit your condition, you can ask your GP to assess you first, investigate the problem if necessary and direct you to the most appropriate practitioner. If you see a physical therapist directly, a qualified practitioner should be able to assess whether they can help you, or whether you need medical investigation.

I refer many patients for various physical therapies and I have tried a lot of them myself at one time or another. In most cases there is no cut and dried formula for the right type of therapy. It is a matter of diagnosing what is causing the problem, having an understanding of each therapy, and then referring to the one most likely to be able to treat the underlying cause of your symptoms. Some people respond well to one type of therapy, while another person with what appears to be the same condition will find a different type of treatment works best for them.

The other factor that comes into play is that with any manual therapy, some practitioners will be more skilled than others. For example, as a health consumer, I have found that one physiotherapist might be ineffective while another physiotherapist with the same qualifications will be able to fix the problem. The same goes for other types of practitioners.

In terms of making decisions about what therapy is best for you, it is often a case of trying out different treatments and practitioners to see what works.

PHYSIOTHERAPY

I often refer to physiotherapists for management of sports injuries and to assist in the management of respiratory problems such as asthma, bronchitis and emphysema.

Physiotherapy originally started out as a hospital practice to help patients recover from surgery, stroke or major injury and restore their normal function. Physiotherapists treat a range of musculoskeletal problems and injuries.

Some physiotherapists specialise into areas such as sports injury treatment and prevention, arthritis, incontinence, brain injury rehabilitation, neck and back problems and more. Chest physiotherapy and lung rehabilitation can help in the treatment of asthma and emphysema.

Physiotherapists are university educated, trained to work out the underlying causes of joint, muscle and nerve injuries, and provide treatment to ensure that people can resume their normal activities as soon as possible. They differ in how much hands-on treatment they provide. Usually they offer a combination of massage, gentle manipulation, stretching, some machinery – interferential and ultrasound – exercise and education in movement and posture.

OSTEOPATHY

Osteopathy can be effective for back pain and neck pain – but not disc prolapse – as well as migraine and other types of headache. Evidence is limited as to whether osteopathic techniques are effective in other conditions.

Osteopathy focuses on the link between the structure of the body and the way it functions. Diagnosis will involve assessment of restrictions in joint movements, areas of tension and tightness in muscles, and problems in the connective tissues under the skin. Therapists also consider the circulation, nervous system and lymphatic system. During your assessment you will be questioned about your symptoms, medical history, lifestyle and diet, and then asked to undress down to your underwear and carry out movements such as sitting, bending over, standing or walking.

The osteopath will then use a combination of soft tissue massage, stretching, mobilisation and manipulation techniques. They will give advice on posture, movement and exercise.

Osteopaths in Australia are university trained and fall under a national registration scheme that ensures professional standards.

CHIROPRACTIC

Chiropractic involves the treatment of the neuromuscular system and can be beneficial in treating lower back pain, neck pain and some causes of headache. It involves manual therapy, particularly manipulation of the spine, joints and soft tissues.

In a chiropractic consultation you will be asked for a description of your symptoms and your medical history. Your posture and movement will be examined. You will be asked to lie down on the treatment bed and the chiropractor will perform a number of short, quick manipulations of different parts of your spine. You may hear a cracking sound like the noise you hear when you crack your knuckles. The aim is to increase the range of motion of the respective joints.

It is less certain whether the chiropractic explanation, that the origin of most illnesses is related to spinal malalignment, is accurate, or whether chiropractic is effective for many other conditions for which it is commonly used. A minority of chiropractors claim that vertebral subluxations – joints in the spine that are out of alignment – are the cause of disease. This is the source of the controversy over chiropractic that you may have heard. There is no scientific evidence to support this claim, and the majority of chiropractors have distanced themselves from this view.

Precautions: one extensive research review found that the risk of neck manipulation outweighed the benefits. At this stage I advise against chiropractic neck manipulation for this reason, although some chiropractors would consider this a conservative position to take.

MASSAGE

Massage can be beneficial for a wide range of physical and psychological conditions and symptoms, including:

- *stress relief*
- *pain management*
- *injury*
- *anxiety and depression*
- *tension headache*
- *back pain due to muscle tension*
- *circulation problems*
- *joint stiffness.*

There are dozens of different forms of massage, but they can be broadly categorised into therapeutic massage and relaxation massage. All massage techniques involve using pressure to encourage blood flow to muscles and connective tissues.

The type of massage you choose will depend on the effect you want. If you want to relax and ease anxiety, then you will be looking for a type of relaxation massage.

The different types of therapeutic, or remedial, massage include:

- **Swedish or 'therapeutic' massage** – *designed to relax muscles and improve circulation*

- **acupressure massage** – *based on the principles of acupuncture*

- **tui na massage** – *an integral part of TCM and is taught in TCM schools as part of formal training in Oriental medicine. The practitioner may brush, knead, roll or press, and rub the areas between each of the joints to get the energy moving in the meridians and the muscles*

- **Thai** – *Thai massage involves stretching and deep massage. This form of bodywork is usually performed on the floor, wearing comfortable clothes that allow for movement. No oils are used in Thai massage. It is known in Thailand as 'nuad phaen thai'*

- **Ayurvedic** – *originating from India, Ayurvedic massage forms a part of Ayurvedic tradition*

- **shiatsu** – *Japanese for finger pressure, which consists of finger and hand pressure and stretching*

- **trigger point therapy** – *focusing on treatment of tight knots of muscle fibres causing pain*
- **Lomi Lomi** – *traditional Hawaiian massage, part of traditional Hawaiian healing practice*
- **stone massage** – *heated smooth, flat stones are placed on key points on the body and sometimes used to massage large muscle areas*
- **lymphatic massage** – *a gentle, superficial form of massage designed to improve lymphatic flow and reduce fluid retention.*

When you have a massage you will be asked to remove some or all of your clothes but usually you keep your underpants on, and any areas of your body not being massaged at a particular time will be covered with towels. You should be asked if there is any part of your body you do not want to be massaged. Usually the therapist will use oil with or without aromatherapy essential oils.

Precautions: do not have massage if you have a bleeding disorder, a thrombosis, are taking blood thinners or if you have a fever.

REFLEXOLOGY

Many claims are made for the health benefits of reflexology; however, at this stage research into this therapy is very limited and scientific evidence has not demonstrated any benefit above and beyond a regular foot massage by someone with no reflexology training.

Reflexology is a form of foot massage. Its philosophy is based on the premise that there are 'reflex' points on the feet that correspond to a structure or organ elsewhere in the body. The therapy relies on a combination of massage and pressure to different points on your feet with the aim of stimulating physiological changes in these organs to encourage the body's own healing potential.

If you have a reflexology treatment, do not expect it to be like a gentle foot massage. The idea is that the greater the area of tenderness, the more likely there is to be a problem in the corresponding area of the body.

Reflexologists are not qualified to diagnose or treat specific medical conditions and if there is any suggestion of a medical problem, you will need to see your doctor to confirm or exclude a diagnosis. If you have foot problems like corns, calluses, bunions, ingrowing toenails or painful feet, then you need to see a podiatrist rather than a reflexologist.

MOVING FORWARD

YOUR GOALS

Goal	Activity	Obstacles/solutions	Result
Reduce reliance on pain killers for neck pain and reduce neck pain	Acupuncture	Making the time and checking the qualifications of the practitioner: see my GP for acupuncture treatments	Reduced pain and reduced use of pain killers

TAKING THE RIGHT PHARMACEUTICAL DRUGS

Here's a scenario I see all the time.

Me: 'Good morning, I am Dr Phelps.'

Patient: 'Hello, Doctor. I have come to see you because I am just feeling awful lately and we can't figure out what's wrong.'

Me: 'Tell me about any medications you are taking.'

Patient: 'Well, there's one of those little blue pills and a half of one of the white blood pressure pills in the morning.'

Me: 'That's all then?'

Patient: 'Yes, that's it. I was on some other pink blood pressure pills but they weren't working so I got changed to the white one about three months ago.'

Me: 'Any other medications? What about supplements or natural therapies?'

Patient: 'Oh yes. I have this brown liquid that smells and tastes revolting but it's supposed to be really good for your adrenals. I take that twice, sometimes three times a day when I remember; some vitamin C and garlic and this other green herbal tablet I get from the health food store when I get a cold. Oh, and a natural sleepy thing for when I can't get off to sleep. Starts with a "V", I think.'

Me: 'Do you have any of these with you or do you have the doses written down? The prescriptions for the pharmacy maybe? No?'

While this example may sound extreme, I can assure you it's a surprisingly common scenario. You might think that as long as your medication is in its original labelled packets and you remember to take it at the right times, there's not so much need to know the details. Well actually, there is. It is important to know exactly what you are taking and why, including prescribed drugs, supplements, vitamins and herbal medicines. You need to know details like the brand name, the generic name, dose, how often it is taken and any special instructions like whether it should be taken before food or with meals.

It is also essential to keep an updated written record in your wallet. This is necessary if you see any practitioner, or if you are asked by a pharmacist about medicines. If you are admitted to hospital for elective surgery, some drugs and supplements may interfere with anaesthetic agents or delay surgery because of their impact on bleeding times. If you are taken to hospital in an emergency, an accurate account of the medications you are taking is extremely important information that might impact on the diagnosis or on aspects of the treatment you receive.

There are broader issues of safety with medications, too. While the right medication taken correctly can save your life or greatly improve your quality of life, medication errors and adverse effects are responsible for a huge amount of misery and a significant number of deaths. Studies have shown that more than 140,000 Australians are admitted to hospital every year as a result of problems with the use of medicines, including adverse reactions.

From my perspective in general practice, a 'fine-tooth comb' review of medications is a routine part of any health assessment. We often discover that a medication or supplement, or a combination, a patient is taking is the reason they are feeling unwell, rather than getting the improved health they sought from taking the medication. Some examples of this are the heightened anxiety people can feel as a side effect of prescribed antidepressants, or the sleeplessness some people experience if they take excessive doses of B group vitamins.

Here is another important reason to understand as much as you can about your medication. You need to read the consumer literature about side effects so that you can recognise if your health problem or new symptoms could be medication-related. This will be available either through your pharmacist, or from the official website of the pharmaceutical company that produced the medication, or government-approved websites.

One of the outcomes I see with medication reviews is that we discover there is no need for medication at all, or the need has long passed but the medication has been continued. This happens a lot with antidepressant medication, where it might have been prescribed many years earlier for a single episode of depression or a period of emotional trauma, and the medication continues to be listed as a regular treatment on the patient's record and repeat prescriptions are rolled over indefinitely without a trial off medication. It can also happen with blood pressure medication after lifestyle changes have reduced the need for the previous doses or eliminated the need for medication at all.

In these days of instant gratification and 'a pill for every ill' mentality, it can be easy to fall into the trap of taking:

- *a medication you can do without*
- *the wrong medication*

- *the right medication for too long or not long enough*
- *medication in the wrong dose or in the wrong combinations.*

Medication errors of all sorts can make you feel pretty ordinary or pretty awful, and they can even be life threatening.

Adverse drug reactions

- Each year in Australia, about 17.5 million people make about 96 million visits to their GP.
- Based on an estimate that 10.4 per cent of patients attending general practice experience an adverse drug event (ADE), almost 2 million people have an ADE annually.
- These ADEs are not trivial, with about 1 million being moderate or severe, and 138,000 requiring hospitalisation. Many of these ADEs are preventable, although the exact proportion of preventable events can be debated.

Adverse drug reactions and interactions are scarily common. Literally millions of them are reported every year. Some reactions will be mild and reasonably benign, like nausea or an upset stomach and once you stop the medication, the side effect goes away, so if it is just a short course it is worth persisting with the medication. Some reactions, like allergic rashes, can be an indication that a more serious allergic reaction could occur in the future.

More severe reactions end up causing a hospitalisation. This could be an anaphylaxis, a severe allergy, or it might be a bleed in the gut, severe anxiety, headaches, gut inflammation or a multitude of other potential problems.

It is very possible that the reason you are feeling less well than you could is because the medication or supplements or the combination you are taking is causing a side effect that you do not realise is an adverse reaction to the medication. Maybe you are not taking the right medication, or you do not need medication at all.

Sometimes medications interfere with the absorption of essential vitamins and minerals from food, leading to micronutrient deficiencies.

One example is the magnesium deficiency that is a common side effect of proton pump inhibitors prescribed to lower stomach acid or treat gastro-oesophageal reflux. This could be the reason you are feeling tired or anxious or not sleeping, you are putting on weight or losing weight, you have constipation or diarrhoea, or you are just feeling a bit off colour.

I am not just referring to the short-term effects of medication within hours or days. Some medications are being reassessed for their dangerous long-term effects. Just a few recent examples are:

- *osteoporosis caused by SSRI (selective serotonin reuptake inhibitor) antidepressants*
- *increased breast cancer rates in women taking long-term hormone replacement therapy*
- *jaw necrosis in some patients taking long-term bisphosphonate medication for osteoporosis*
- *coenzyme Q10 deficiency if you are taking statins to lower cholesterol*
- *vitamin B_{12} deficiency and magnesium deficiency in people taking long-term acid suppression medicine called proton pump inhibitors (PPIs).*

Safe use of medicines

- ❧ Have your medicines and supplements reviewed with your GP at least once a year. If you no longer need to take a medication, ask for advice on how to safely reduce the dose or cease it, or whether there is a safe or effective natural medicine or lifestyle modification that could replace it.
- ❧ If you are seeing a new GP, take along all the bottles and packets of medication and supplements you are taking, including those you take only occasionally. This is the only way to get a completely accurate account of what is going on in your body chemistry.
- ❧ Check all the labels for ingredients and do an internet search of the medical literature to see if the health problems you have could be related to any of your medications.
- ❧ Check the correct dose of the medication, how often it should be taken, and whether you need to take it with food or before or after meals. Also check the use-by date on the packet.
- ❧ Before you start taking any new medicine, double check for any adverse effects or potential interactions with other drugs or herbal medicines or supplements.

- Record and report any allergic reactions to any medication.
- Check whether any medicine you are taking or plan to take is safe with alcohol.
- Find out if the medicine needs to be kept refrigerated. Examples of this are thyroxine for the treatment of underactive thyroid, and most probiotic formulations.
- The same advice applies to herbal therapies. Do not just keep taking the same preparation you were once prescribed without reassessment of your current needs.
- Go through your home medicine cabinet regularly and dispose of any out-of-date medicines. You can take them to your pharmacist or GP, who will safely dispose of them for you.
- If you take a number of medicines, your pharmacist can arrange special packaging of all your medications to reduce the risk of missing doses or doubling up.
- Pay special attention if you are pregnant or likely to become pregnant while you are taking any medication.
- Do not take medications prescribed for someone else and do not offer your medication to someone else, even if you think they have the same condition.

HERBAL MEDICINE

As part of your plan to achieve ultimate wellbeing, you may consider taking herbs. You might take herbal medicines either on their own, instead of pharmaceutical medicines or in addition to pharmaceutical. There is some important information for you to know about taking herbal preparations, particularly the safety of a herb or supplement if you are trying to get pregnant, undergoing cancer treatment or planning surgery.

For thousands of years, herbs and plants found in their natural environment have formed the foundation of remedies used in traditional medical systems around the world, including the health practices of Ancient Egypt and Ancient Greece, indigenous Australian healing practices, the Ayurvedic tradition in India, TCM and European herbal medicine.

Many of the commonly used pharmaceutical products in Western medical practice today were based on traditional plant remedies such as aspirin (from meadowsweet), digoxin (from *Digitalis purpurea*), ephedrine (from *Ephedra sineca*), colchicine (from autumn crocus), morphine (from *Papaver somniferum*) and the chemotherapy drug vincristine (from Madagascar periwinkle). Herbs, unlike pharmaceutical products, are not a single chemical substance. They are in fact chemically complex with multiple constituents and functions, and interactions within the human body.

What to stop and when, before surgery

When there is a concern about blood loss or bleeding times with surgery, you will need to get advice on whether to stop taking high doses of concentrated supplements – not food sources – of the 'G' herbs five to seven days before surgery: garlic, ginger, ginkgo biloba and ginseng.

Despite millennia of traditional use, detailed scientific testing is relatively new to the study of herbal medicine. Some herbs have been shown to be extremely effective and safe in the treatment of specific conditions. Research has also started to give us some detail about which herbs, doses and combinations work for specific conditions and where we might need to warn people of the potential for adverse effects or interactions with other herbs or drugs.

Pharmaceutical-grade extracts are not interchangeable with their naturally occurring relatives. There are very significant differences you need to know about in order to understand how herbs work and how to use them safely in the context of your health. The complexity of herbs and the nature of medical research methods make it very tempting for scientists involved in pharmaceutical development to try to identify and isolate a single active ingredient in a herb. This ignores the fact that in many cases, it is the very complexity of the herb that is responsible for the way it works when it is used as a medicine. While there may be one or several active ingredients, other constituents might influence the way those 'actives' are absorbed, distributed in the body, metabolised and ultimately excreted by your body.

Think about the fruit and vegetables you buy at the local market or supermarket: they are all products of nature, but the flavour and quality vary markedly with the season and growing conditions, including the location of farms, soil quality, rainfall, environmental temperatures, storage methods and other factors. Herbs are also products of nature and will vary somewhat depending on these factors as well as the precise species of herb, the part of the plant used, and the harvesting and processing method.

A herbal product might be sourced from leaves, stems, fruit, flowers, seeds, roots, rhizomes – an underground stem such as ginger – or bark. Preparations can be in the form of raw herbs, tinctures, liquid extracts, syrups, tablets, capsules or creams. Some herbal medicines come packaged and labelled, others are sold as raw herbs to be made into tea. All liquid preparations prescribed and mixed individually should be obtained only from a qualified herbal medicine practitioner.

Good suppliers and manufacturers try to standardise their products as much as possible with chemical analysis and quality control at all stages of production, but some poorer quality products may contain few or none of the active ingredients you think you are buying.

You might be struck by the variation in cost of some of the herbal preparations compared with others that may seem equivalent in content. That is not to say that because one brand or preparation is vastly more expensive than another that it must essentially be superior, but it is a reason to ask some questions about the quality of the product. It is also a reason not to assume that a different brand of herbal medicine will give you equivalent results to one you have tried before.

I have seen patients who started out getting good clinical results with their first course or two of a herbal medicine, only to find the effect 'wore off'. On closer questioning, the effect did not 'wear off' at all, but they had bought a different brand at a discount supplier or over the internet, expecting it to be the same because the name of the herb on the label was the same. All of those other factors, such as the soil the plant was grown in, the processing method, the amount of active ingredients, and the presence of contaminants may be factors.

REGULATIONS FOR QUALITY AND SAFETY

Regulations concerning the manufacture and sale of herbs differ from country to country. In Australia there is strict government regulation overseen by the Therapeutic Goods Administration (TGA). All herbal products manufactured commercially in Australia must be produced according to the code of Good Manufacturing Practice (GMP), and they are listed (L) or registered (R) with an AUST L or AUST R rating. You will see one of these terms on the label with a number following it.

Most herbal medicines, most vitamin and mineral supplements, other nutritional supplements, traditional medicines such as Ayurvedic medicines and traditional Chinese medicines, and aromatherapy oils have an AUST L rating, which means they are considered low risk and generally safe, contain only permitted ingredients and conform to good manufacturing standards.

An AUST R rating applies to a very small number of complementary medicines where the TGA has been satisfied that specific claims of efficacy in treatment or prevention of a disease are supported by adequate evidence.

Aside from strict manufacturing standards, manufacturers also have strict regulations about labelling and advertising.

- *In the USA, since 1994 the FDA (Food and Drug Administration) has classified herbal medicines as foods. Manufacturers are responsible for product safety and they are removed from the market only if there is found to be a safety risk to consumers.*

- *In Canada, herbal medicines are classified as 'natural health products' and products have to be reviewed and obtain a licence before they go to market.*

- *In Germany, herbal medicines have always been an integral part of mainstream medical practice and you need a prescription to obtain them.*

- *In the UK, some herbs need a medical prescription, some have to be registered as Traditional Herbal Medicinal Products, while others have free rein to be used as foods or supplements.*

> From country to country, herbal medicines are treated differently, with some countries insisting on medical prescription, some having a form of regulated over-the-counter sale, and others where there is little regulation and herbal medicines are simply sold as foods or dietary supplements or incorporated into 'functional foods'.

Generally speaking, herbal medicines that are processed and used properly are considered very safe, but side effects and interactions can and do happen. This is particularly important to consider because herbal medicine preparations are so widely available without professional advice, and people commonly self-medicate for various reasons, such as to increase their energy levels, boost immunity, fend off colds and flu, relieve pain or improve symptoms that cannot be easily defined. While you might get it right, there are pitfalls.

If you are considering taking a herbal medicine, I would highly recommend seeking professional advice rather than trying to figure it out yourself and risk taking the wrong type of preparation or the wrong dose or both.

If your doctor does not know much about herbal medicines, or worse, gives you a hard time because you mention it, you may need to find a new doctor who has some experience with herbal medicines or is open to working with a qualified herbalist.

(See the chapter 'Choosing the Right Health Professionals' on page 34.)

TEN WAYS TO SAFE DECISIONS ABOUT HERBAL MEDICINE

- *Be clear on what you are hoping to achieve using herbal medicine. Do you want to stay well? Improve your energy? Relieve a symptom? Counteract the side effects of a medical treatment like chemotherapy? Prevent illness? Reduce the need for pharmaceutical medication?*

- Consider the therapeutic options singly or in combination:
  - *lifestyle changes*
  - *medical intervention*
  - *herbal medicines*
  - *other natural therapies.*
- *If you choose a herbal medicine option, check what herb(s) are in a preparation, as they are often in combination.*
- *Preferably get trained professional advice on the correct dose and combination for your particular condition. Make sure you inform the practitioner about all of your other medications and supplements, including over-the-counter and prescription items. When you see your GP, make sure you tell them exactly what herbal preparations you are taking as they might be important in your medical history. Where Chinese herbs are involved, definitely see a qualified and preferably registered TCM practitioner.*
- *Ask questions and read up about the benefits and risks associated with the herbal medicine, including potential drug interactions.*
- *Select quality products, checking there is an AUST L or AUST R number and an expiry date on the product label; or, if the product comes from overseas, make sure it is manufactured according to the Code of Good Manufacturing Practice.*
- *Buy the product from a reputable source. Internet purchases are notoriously unreliable.*
- *Ask how long you can expect to take the preparation before you notice an effect. This might vary from under an hour to several weeks or months.*
- *Report any possible adverse reactions to your doctor or prescriber, the manufacturer, and the relevant herbal and natural medicine associations.*
- *If you add any new drugs or supplements while you are taking the herbal medicine, let your pharmacist or health professional know to make sure the combination is safe.*

MY LIST OF SOME HERBS WORTH KNOWING ABOUT

This is not an exhaustive list, but these common herbs are useful and widely available. I have listed the most usual reasons for prescription to begin each entry, so you can assess quickly how relevant the information on this herb may be to you.

It is important to bear in mind that herbs are very often prescribed in combination with other herbs to enhance their effect. Some herbs will also interact with prescribed and over the counter medications, so if you are taking medicines, and particularly if you have a significant medical problem, you will need to exercise special caution and ask for professional advice. You may be able to reduce the number of pharmaceuticals you take, or their doses, but this should be managed in consultation with your GP.

The purpose of this list is to give you an idea of the breadth of uses for herbal medicines and some of the precautions to consider before you decide to take them, particularly if you are self-prescribing (which I would discourage). The herbs included in this list are some of the ones I find most useful in general practice, or ones that I am frequently asked about by patients. I have deliberately not included doses because different preparations have different dosage levels and the instructions on the label or professional advice need to be carefully followed.

If you are pregnant, or are likely to become pregnant, you will need professional advice before taking a herb. One of the problems is that herbal medicines have generally not been tested for safety in pregnancy, so caution is advised. While it is rarely a cause for alarm if you do happen to get pregnant while you are taking a herbal medicine, you will usually be advised to stop that herb unless it has specific evidence of safety in pregnancy or during breastfeeding. One notable exception to this is ginger, which is used for treating nausea in pregnancy.

Andrographis (andrographis paniculata *or King of Bitters*)

Prescribed for:

- *preventing colds in winter months*

- *helping with the symptoms of common viral respiratory infections*

- *boosting immunity*

Andrographis is widely used in the traditional medicine of India, China and Korea. I find it very useful in general practice for helping with the symptoms of common viral respiratory infections. Obviously antibiotics are not useful for these, so a herbal medicine that relieves symptoms within a few days comes in very handy. It is also used at lower doses to prevent colds in winter months.

Andrographis is often used in combination with Siberian ginseng as a tonic to assist in recuperation. Used with peppermint, it also aids appetite and digestion.

Tablet form is the best way to take this, as it is very bitter as a liquid.

Precautions:

There are some drug interactions, particularly immunosuppressants, blood thinners and oral diabetes drugs, so check before you take it.

It should be ceased a week before major surgery because of its anti-blood-clotting activity.

Astragalus

Prescribed for:

- *stimulating immunity*
- *recovering from viral infection*
- *stress relief*
- *chronic kidney disease*
- *improving heart function in cardiovascular disease*
- *protecting the liver*
- *reducing side effects of cancer chemotherapy.*

Astragalus has been known to TCM for thousands of years, and in herbal medicine is referred to as an 'adaptogen', a natural substance with the ability to help the body to cope with, or adapt to, physical and emotional stresses. It is best known as an immune stimulant, and also for its antioxidant properties, to improve heart function in cardiovascular disease and to protect the liver. Astragalus is commonly used to prevent colds and flu, and to aid in recuperation from viral infections.

In TCM it is also prescribed to treat chronic kidney disease.

It has a slight oestrogen-like effect and this is why it is sometimes included in menopause treatment.

Astragalus is commonly prescribed for cancer patients to enhance the effectiveness and reduce the side effects of chemotherapy.

Precautions:

At recommended doses, astragalus is well tolerated but it may interact with drugs or other herbs; specifically, immunosuppressants and lithium.

It appears to lower blood sugar, so if you are on diabetes medication your blood sugar levels will need to be monitored.

In TCM, astragalus is not used to treat the acute phase of an infection.

If you are using astragulus while undergoing chemotherapy for cancer treatment, your cancer specialist will need to know.

Bilberry (Vaccinium myrtillus)

Prescribed for:

- *strengthening blood vessels and improving circulation*
- *preventing and treating diabetic retinal problems*
- *improving poor night vision*
- *acute diarrhoea*
- *topical treatment for mild inflammation in the mouth and throat.*

Compounds called anthocyanosides strengthen blood vessels and improve circulation. Bilberry is related to blueberry and has strong antioxidant properties. Research is underway to see if it is able to slow the formation of cataracts.

Precautions:

Bilberry fruit and extract are considered safe, but the bilberry leaf and leaf extract should not be taken at high doses or over a long period of time because it can cause severe weight loss and muscle spasms, and can be fatal.

At very high doses it might interfere with warfarin and other anti-clotting drugs.

Bilberry appears to lower blood sugar, so if you are on diabetes medication your blood sugar levels will need to be monitored.

Black cohosh (Cimicifuga racemosa *or* Actea racemosa)

Prescribed for:

- *menopausal symptoms like hot flushes, irritability and vaginal dryness*
- *premenstrual syndrome.*

This is a very popular herbal medicine in women's health, particularly since research raised serious concerns about the risk of hormone replacement therapy for menopausal and perimenopausal women. It won't work for every woman, but it is effective in a significant number of women who are troubled by menopausal symptoms like hot flushes, irritability and vaginal dryness. Black cohosh might take a few weeks to a few months to work. It is frequently used in combination with other herbs such as St John's wort if more of a mood-stabilising effect is needed.

In Europe it is also recommended for treatment of premenstrual syndrome and period pain. It can help treat menstrual migraine.

Precautions:

If you are having treatment for breast cancer, your specialist will need to know if you are taking black cohosh because it might increase the activity and effectiveness of some types of chemotherapy.

Adverse side effects are rare but might include headache and dizziness, and there have been rare isolated reports of liver damage.

Calendula (marigold)

Prescribed for:

- *antibacterial and anti-inflammatory action*
- *accelerating wound healing*
- *treating burns.*

This is one for your household medicine cabinet. Calendula cream has antibacterial and anti-inflammatory effects and is great for accelerating wound healing. It also works very well as a burn cream, and as a topical treatment for skin inflammation, bruises, boils, cracked nipples, sunburn and nappy rash.

Calendula has a soothing effect on skin burns from radiotherapy.

Precautions:

Calendula is considered to be very safe. There are occasional reports of allergic reactions. No interactions with other drugs or herbs are known.

Chaste tree (Vitex agnus castus)

Prescribed for:

- *a variety of women's health issues including infrequent or irregular periods, heavy periods and premenstrual syndrome*
- *hormonal breast pain*
- *enhancing fertility.*

Like most female doctors, I see a lot of patients with gynaecological problems. I must say, I find this herb is among the most useful ones for a variety of women's health issues including infrequent or irregular periods, heavy periods and premenstrual syndrome. It relieves PMS symptoms including irritability, breast tenderness, headaches and constipation. It can also relieve perimenopausal and menopausal symptoms and reduce fibroids.

It may help in the treatment of hormone-related acne.

Chaste tree helps to improve fertility in women related to hormone imbalance, particularly progesterone deficiency.

The most consistent extract has the code Ze440.

In breastfeeding it is used to increase milk supply.

Precautions:

Any unexplained heavy menstrual bleeding or menstrual irregularity needs to be medically investigated prior to any treatment decisions.

Cranberry (Vaccinium macrocarpon)

Prescribed for:

- *prevention of recurring urinary tract infections.*

Cranberry is available as juice or as tablets. The juice is widely available but if you don't like the taste, or if you don't want the extra calories from the juice, the tablet form might suit you better.

It can also be used to deodorise urine in cases of urinary incontinence.

Precautions:

Diabetics should use the tablet form rather than the juice because of the sugar content of the juice.

Established urinary tract infections need to be treated medically to avoid kidney complications.

If you are taking warfarin, your doses need to be checked when you start taking cranberry.

Devil's claw (Harpagophytum procumbens)

Prescribed for:

- *anti-inflammatory and analgesic effects*
- *symptom relief for osteoarthritis and lower back pain.*

Precautions:

Because it can increase stomach acid, do not take devil's claw if you have a history of peptic ulcer or gallstones. You will need medical advice if you are taking blood thinning medication or medications for diabetes.

Echinacea (Echinacea angustifolia *and* Echinacea purpurea)

Prescribed for:

- *boosting immunity*
- *treating acute viral respiratory infections such as colds and sinusitis*
- *as an antifungal and antibacterial*
- *acne*

- *herpes infections*
- *candida (in conjunction with antifungal medication).*

Precautions:

There have been some reports of allergic reactions. Caution is advised if you are taking immunosuppressant drugs, particularly cyclophosphamide and cyclosporine.

Evening primrose oil (Oenothera biennis)

I thought I would include evening primrose oil (EPO) on this list as much for what it can't do as for what it can do. It was a common perception that EPO was an effective treatment for premenstrual syndrome and menopausal flushes, and a lot of my female patients would come to see me for advice after trying EPO on the suggestion of a friend or something they had read. When EPO was formally tested it was found to be ineffective. In the case of menopause, it can even make hot flushes worse.

EPO might help some women with breast pain as their main premenstrual problem, but the effect is usually minor.

EPO has been shown to reduce the symptoms of endometriosis. It helps treat nerve damage from diabetes (diabetic neuropathy). It has an anti-inflammatory pain-relieving effect in rheumatoid arthritis.

Precautions:

EPO should be suspended for a week before surgery. There are some drug interactions, including blood thinners and phenothiazines used to treat schizophrenia. It should be used with caution in people with some forms of epilepsy; for example, temporal lobe epilepsy.

Feverfew (Tanacetum parthenium)

Prescribed for:

- *fever*
- *headache*
- *arthritis.*

Feverfew is a member of the sunflower family and has traditionally been used as a remedy for fever, headache and arthritis.

In general practice we mainly use feverfew in conjunction with magnesium and riboflavin (vitamin B_2) for the prevention of migraine in patients who want to minimise the use of pharmaceutical medications.

It is possible that some types of preparations are more effective than others.

Side effects:

- *abdominal pain*
- *diarrhoea*
- *nausea*
- *interaction with blood thinners such as warfarin.*

Precautions:

Feverfew should not be used in pregnancy. Allergic reaction can occur in susceptible people. If you take feverfew for longer than a week, do not stop taking it abruptly because you can get a discontinuation effect, including headache, anxiety and fatigue.

Garlic (Allium sativum)

Prescribed for:

- *lowering blood pressure*
- *slowing the progression of atherosclerosis (hardening of the arteries)*
- *antithrombotic (anti-clotting effects) on blood*
- *relieving symptoms of the common cold.*

Garlic is a food and a medicine. It can be used fresh, both raw or cooked, or taken in capsules or tablets, or as an oil.

It is an antioxidant. Garlic can slightly lower blood pressure and slow the progression of atherosclerosis. It has an antithrombotic effect on blood. Although it has been thought to lower cholesterol, evidence does not support this.

Garlic has an antibacterial and antiviral effect, and is used to relieve symptoms of the common cold. It also has an antifungal effect, and can be used to treat tinea infections.

Side effects:

The main problems with garlic is that it can cause bad breath, heartburn and upset stomach, so enteric-coated odourless preparations are usually better tolerated and more socially acceptable.

Precautions:

Garlic is safe for most people. Do not take garlic as a medicine without medical advice if you have a clotting or bleeding disorder, or diabetes.

Garlic has been found to interfere with the effectiveness of the anti-HIV drugs saquinavir and ritonavir.

Stop high dose supplements a week before surgery or dental work. Garlic does not appear to affect warfarin.

Allergic reactions are possible.

Ginger (Zingiber officinalis)

Prescribed for:

- *prevention and treatment of motion sickness*
- *increasing appetite*
- *relieving the nausea of cancer chemotherapy*
- *lowering blood pressure*
- *lowering blood sugar*
- *pregnancy-associated nausea.*

Apart from its use in cooking, ginger has long been used in Asian, Indian and Arabic herbal traditions.

Precautions:

Don't take ginger as a herbal medicine without medical advice if you have gallstones, a bleeding or clotting disorder, or if you are on medication for diabetes or high blood pressure.

Ginkgo (Ginkgo biloba)

Prescribed for:

- *improving blood flow, so we use it to improve circulation in the legs and to relieve chilblains*
- *relieving the symptoms of Raynaud's syndrome*
- *countering the sexual dysfunction associated with some antidepressant drugs*
- *relieving breast tenderness and irritability in premenstrual syndrome*
- *preventing altitude sickness.*

Ginkgo is extremely popular in Europe and is one of the top herbal medicines used in France and Germany, for a multitude of uses.

The most extensively studied extract has the code EGb 761.

There has been a lot of hype about the promise of ginkgo biloba in the treatment of dementia. Unfortunately, while a number of studies have shown improvements in memory, thinking and behaviour in people with early stage dementia, it does not seem to slow the progression of the disease. And larger studies on ginkgo and dementia prevention have shown disappointing results.

Precautions:

Stop taking ginkgo one week before major surgery.

Green tea (Camellia sinensis)

This is a fascinating plant with a myriad of health benefits. It has a high antioxidant content.

Prescribed for:

- *reducing LDL-cholesterol or 'bad cholesterol'*
- *reducing stroke risk*
- *helping with weight loss because it reduces appetite and boosts metabolism*
- *reducing blood sugar levels.*

Research suggests it may provide some cancer protective effects. It can reduce inflammation in inflammatory bowel disease, such as Crohn's disease, and may protect the liver against toxins like excessive alcohol.

Green tea comes from the same plant as black tea and oolong tea, but is processed differently and contains less caffeine.

Precautions:

Tannins in tea can reduce iron absorption, so green tea preferably should not be drunk within two hours of a meal. There are some drug interactions.

Hawthorn (Crataegus oxycantha)

Prescribed for:

- *positive effects on heart function*
- *increasing coronary blood flow*
- *reducing the heart muscle's need for oxygen*
- *stabilising heart rhythm and pulse rate*
- *lowering blood pressure.*

Precautions:

If you have symptoms of heart disease, such as chest pain, breathlessness or swollen ankles, it is essential to seek medical advice and be treated under careful medical supervision.

This herb should never be self-prescribed or used in cases where you have not been medically diagnosed and treated.

Horse chestnut (Aesculus hippocastanum)

Prescribed for:

- *oedema (fluid swelling)*
- *inflammation in the legs due to chronic venous insufficiency*
- *varicose veins and venous leg ulcers.*

Usually the seed of the plant relieves pain and swelling in the legs after about three to 12 weeks of treatment. It can be used orally and topically for treatment of haemorrhoids, where it takes six days to work.

Side effects:

- *stomach upset*
- *skin irritation*
- *dizziness*
- *nausea*
- *headache.*

Horse chestnut should be taken after food to avoid stomach upset. People who are allergic to latex may also be allergic to horse chestnut.

Precautions:

May reduce blood sugar levels so can interact with oral diabetes drugs.

Lavender (Lavandula angustifolia)

Prescribed for:

- *Relaxation.*

The scent of lavender is a very familiar perfume, and aside from its use in soaps and cosmetics it has a long history in herbal medicine. Lavender scent from a diffuser has a relaxing effect, and has been shown to help settle elderly people with dementia and agitation.

Here's a useful tip: lavender has also been shown to calm dogs that suffer from travel-induced overexcitement.

Marshmallow (Althaea officinalis)

Prescribed for:

- *Soothing mucous membranes.*

Do you hear the word 'marshmallow' and immediately think of fluffy white sugary balls on the end of a stick roasting on a campfire? The herbal medicine 'marshmallow' is not the same thing. It is an extract from a plant whose roots and leaves are mixed with water to form a gel that coats the throat and stomach, soothing irritated mucous membranes.

Precautions:

Like slippery elm, marshmallow coats the lining of the stomach and gut so you need to separate doses from other herbs or drugs by at least two hours to avoid it affecting their absorption.

Peppermint (Mentha piperita)

Prescribed for:

- *irritable bowel syndrome (IBS)*
- *dyspepsia.*

Peppermint is popularly taken as a herbal tea and in capsules.

Precautions:

Do not take peppermint oil if you have gall bladder inflammation or liver disease.

Rhodiola (Rhodiola rosea)

Prescribed for:

- *anxiety*
- *fatigue*
- *improving mood*
- *depression.*

Rhodiola helps with a rapid response in an extremely stressful situation.

Side effects:

- *dizziness*
- *dry mouth.*

Precautions:

Rhodiola is not recommended in bipolar disorder.

Saw palmetto (Serenoa repens)

Prescribed for:

- *benign prostatic enlargement in men.*

Many older men will be familiar with the symptoms of an enlarged prostate gland, most significantly trouble passing urine. Saw palmetto is a popular herbal remedy, often used in combination with other herbs to relieve the symptoms of benign prostatic hypertrophy. One of its advantages is that it can reduce prostate swelling without altering the prostate specific antigen (PSA) level, the marker for prostate cancer. So if prostate cancer were to develop or worsen, the PSA level would reflect that. You can expect it to take a month or two to show a benefit.

Precautions:

Symptoms of urinary obstruction or infection need to be fully investigated to rule out infection or prostate cancer.

Slippery elm (Ulmus rubra)

Prescribed for:

- *gut problems.*

Slippery elm bark powder is another very useful herbal medicine. We recommend it for relieving the symptoms of a range of gut problems, including gastritis, dyspepsia, gastro-oesophageal reflux, peptic ulcer, irritable bowel syndrome and Crohn's disease.

Precautions:

Slippery elm may interfere with the absorption of some medications, so it is best taken at a different time of the day to medicines that need careful monitoring of dosages, such as digoxin, lithium, warfarin and epilepsy medications.

St John's wort (Hypericum perforatum)

Prescribed for:

- *anxiety*
- *depression*
- *menopausal symptoms.*

St John's wort is a yellow-flowered plant. Its use as a medicine dates back to Ancient Greece where it was used for the treatment of nervous conditions, and it has been used in Europe as a treatment for anxiety and depression since the 1500s. Extensive scientific testing has concluded that it is at least as effective as pharmaceutical antidepressants for the treatment of depression, with fewer side effects. It is also useful for the irritability of premenstrual syndrome and menopause.

The main active constituents are hyperforin and hypericin.

Precautions:

There are multiple potential drug interactions, particularly the SSRI class of antidepressants. Preparations with lower hyperforin content, such as Ze117, are less likely to cause drug interactions.

St Mary's thistle (Silybum marianum)

Prescribed for:

- *liver detox*
- *reducing liver damage.*

St Mary's thistle, also known as milk thistle, is a popular herb used to protect the liver against toxins such as alcohol and medications like paracetamol, and helps to repair liver damage.

Based on traditional use, milk thistle has been used as an antidote to the toxic effects of death cap mushroom.

Siberian ginseng (Eleutherococcus senticosus)

Prescribed for:

- *stimulating immunity*
- *relieving exhaustion or aiding convalescence.*

Siberian ginseng is different from American ginseng or Korean ginseng. It is known as an 'adaptogen', which means it helps the body to adapt to times of emotional and physical stress.

It has an immune stimulating effect and is used to combat fatigue and to increase energy and alertness.

Side effects:

- *increased blood pressure*
- *trouble sleeping*
- *headache*
- *irregular heartbeat.*

Precautions:

Siberian ginseng may interact with a number of medications, including blood thinners, sedatives, diabetes medicines, digoxin, steroids and lithium, so you need to check with your pharmacist or doctor before taking it.

Turmeric (Curcuma longa)

Prescribed for:

- *inflammatory conditions*
- *anticancer effect*
- *antioxidant properties.*

A member of the ginger family, turmeric is grown in India, Asia and Africa, and it is used as a powder or in capsules, teas, or liquid extracts. The active ingredient is curcumin.

Turmeric is thought to have anti-inflammatory, anticancer and antioxidant properties. It is approved in Europe for use in digestive problems. It has been shown to improve remission rates in ulcerative colitis.

Precautions:

Turmeric should be ceased two weeks before surgery. It can interact with blood thinning medications and can lower blood pressure. High doses can cause stomach upset.

Valerian (Valeriana officinalis)

Prescribed for:

- *anxiety*
- *insomnia.*

Valerian is a very popular herbal medicine dating back to the Ancient Greek and Roman physicians Hippocrates and Galen. It is used to relieve anxiety and insomnia, often in combination with other herbs such as passionflower. Some studies have shown it to be as effective as benzodiazepine drugs for people who have trouble falling asleep. It works differently from the benzodiazepines, however, in that it becomes more effective over a couple of weeks of regular use. It does not cause drowsiness the next day and it is not considered to be addictive.

MOVING FORWARD

YOUR GOALS

Goal	Activity	Obstacles/solutions	Result
Reduce anxiety	Take an appropriate dosage of St John's wort	Possible interactions with other treatments: see my GP for advice	Anxiety is lessened

VITAMINS AND NUTRITIONAL SUPPLEMENTS

There is a lot you need to know if you are going to maintain your micronutrients at healthy levels. Of course, the more you can get from fresh foods the better, and from completing your food diary and reading the information in the nutrition chapter you will have a much clearer idea about whether your nutritional needs are being met. But the reality is that most people do not eat a fully balanced, high-quality diet with lots of fresh fruit, vegetables, nuts, whole grains, legumes and the other food groups necessary to get all the elements to keep you in peak shape.

Some conditions such as pregnancy, old age, illness and digestive problems, and factors such as alcohol consumption, taking medications, eating a vegetarian diet and many other situations will make it difficult and perhaps impossible for you to get all the micronutrients. So, if you are feeling less than great, look at the possibility that you are missing one or more essential micronutrients.

Many of them can be tested with simple blood tests (such as iron or vitamin B_{12}), urine tests (for example iodine testing) or a taste test (in the case of zinc deficiency). In other instances, we need to anticipate what the problem might be based on your medical history, any medications you are taking, your current state of health, your diet and any other evidence we can gather.

In some cases, when you replace what is missing you will really feel the difference in the short term. In other cases you will be reducing your risk of longer-term health problems. Beyond simply replacing deficiency, vitamin treatments may be prescribed selectively for a specific treatment effect. In other words, a vitamin or mineral supplement is used as a targeted therapeutic medicine in the same way as a pharmaceutical product might be used.

> If one pill is good, many must be even better, right?

I have seen countless people who arrive with literally a shopping bag full of assorted supplements, but they still feel dreadful and are totally confused about what they should be doing or taking. In some cases, when we total it up, we find they have been taking massively excessive doses of a number of nutrients and copping the side effects rather than the potential for positive effects.

Like many people, you may have dropped by your local pharmacy, health food store or even the supermarket and bought a 'multivitamin', a 'mega B formula', or some sort of 'tonic'. There are a few problems with this approach.

Most importantly, popping a few random vitamin supplements does nothing to address the underlying reasons you are feeling tired or unwell. In addition to that, you can run into problems if you take the wrong supplements, the wrong doses, the wrong combinations, or if you mix them with medications they should not be mixed with.

As just one simple example, I frequently have to advise patients to stop taking huge doses of vitamin B if they find they have become jittery, nervous and sleepless, which are all potential side effects of large doses of B vitamins. I have also seen a number of women around the age of 50 who started taking megadoses of B vitamins because they were feeling fatigued and stressed, then developed what they thought were menopausal hot flushes, when in fact they were getting a niacin flush, a well-known side effect of niacin, or vitamin B_3.

Some drugs that can cause nutrient deficiencies

- ❧ Proton pump inhibitors (PPIs, stomach-acid-lowering medicines): reduce absorption of iron, vitamin B_{12} and folate
- ❧ Diuretics (fluid tablets): increase magnesium loss so increased intake will be needed; cause lower levels of vitamin B_1 and can cause loss of potassium
- ❧ Laxatives: faster bowel transit time may reduce absorption
- ❧ Some antibiotics: reduce vitamin B_{12} levels and vitamin K
- ❧ Drugs to impair fat absorption can cause multiple nutritional deficiencies. One weight loss drug, orlistat, has been shown to reduce the absorption of some fat-soluble vitamins (A, D, E and K) and beta-carotene.

I must make it clear that I am not against taking supplements – far from it. I have seen some near-miraculous recoveries in people who responded to the judicious use of carefully prescribed supplements for a range of micronutrient deficiencies, medical conditions and health states. At my age, I take a selected combination of supplements for health maintenance myself. What I would warn you against is self-diagnosing and then self-prescribing particularly multiple products.

You need to know that vitamins and minerals are chemicals that interact with your own body's chemistry. Pharmaceuticals are also chemicals that interact with your body's chemistry as well as with the other substances you put into your body, including herbs, vitamins, minerals and foods. Some of these interactions will be beneficial to you. But some will have no benefit and some are potentially harmful.

Some pharmaceutical drugs will cause nutrient deficiencies. The major culprits are drugs prescribed to reduce stomach acid, diuretics, laxatives, some antibiotics, drugs that impair fat absorption and some epilepsy drugs. If you are taking any of these, you need to check whether you can get all of the extra nutrients you need through changes in your diet, or whether you need to take a supplement to cover any likely deficiencies.

It is also important not to assume that because something is labelled 'natural' that it is inherently safe under all circumstances.

SPECIAL NEEDS

It is helpful to look at some examples of the groups of people with special needs. If you are in one of these groups, let's look at how you might benefit from nutritional testing and supplementing where necessary.

✤ GETTING OLDER

As you get older, your body becomes less efficient at absorbing the nutrients you need. And your appetite and food intake generally can decrease. If you are living alone, meals can also be monotonous and limited in variety. It is also more likely that with advancing age you may develop a form of chronic disease that will increase your requirements for certain nutrients. Older people are also more likely to be taking one or multiple medications which increases the possibility of interactions.

Vitamin deficiencies are common in elderly people, particularly vitamin A, the B vitamins, vitamin C and vitamin D. The symptoms of deficiency, such as forgetfulness, lack of concentration and fatigue might easily be explained away as the inevitable signs of getting on in years.

❧ PREGNANT WOMEN

If you are pregnant or planning a pregnancy, you need to consider not only your own health and nutritional needs, but also what the baby will need for normal growth and development. Eating a fresh, varied and healthy diet is important during pregnancy, just as it is at any other time.

I think by now you would have to be living under a rock to not know that folate supplements are recommended for every pregnant woman. The use of folate supplements to prevent neural tube defects such as spina bifida is now very well established and supplementation, particularly if you have a poor vegetable intake, with a multivitamin containing 500 micrograms of folate should be started before conception.

More recently, common deficiencies that can affect a foetus have been identified and we recommend testing of iodine and vitamin D levels in pregnant women and supplementation where necessary. Iron, zinc, folate, vitamin D, calcium and iodine are all essential nutrients that may be lacking, and should be included in the choice of a high-quality antenatal supplement. Omega-3 is also recommended for normal foetal brain development.

Some women think that 'if one supplement is good, then more is better', but correct dosing is important. Check the contents of any supplements or over the counter preparations that are being taken, and be sure to avoid excess. This may particularly be the case for substances such as vitamin A.

❧ IF YOU DRINK TOO MUCH ALCOHOL

Alcohol prevents quite a few nutrients from being absorbed. If you drink consistently on most days of the week, or binge drink regularly, there is a high likelihood that you will need to boost your nutrient intake. The most likely deficiencies if you drink heavily are vitamins A, B (including folate), C, D, E and K, and the mineral zinc. There might also be problems with magnesium, calcium and iron.

A good quality multivitamin and mineral is probably the best insurance in this situation. Actually, it is better not to drink too much alcohol, but if you do then you will need to think about your extra nutritional needs.

If you are a regular heavy drinker and you suddenly stop, then you would be wise to talk to your doctor first. High doses of the B group vitamins, especially thiamine and folate, are an important protection against withdrawal symptoms.

✤ IF YOU HAVE DIGESTIVE PROBLEMS

In this chapter on nutrients and supplements you might have noticed there is a lot of mention of digestive problems affecting absorption. There are many reasons why digestion can be less than ideal: chronic diarrhoea, coeliac disease, Crohn's disease and malabsorption problems among them. This might mean your gut is not able to adequately absorb all the vitamins and minerals, fats, proteins and carbohydrates you need, regardless of the quantity of the right foods you eat. In the event of any digestive problems, it is likely that you are going to need to supplement with higher doses of a range of nutrients in order to get the levels you need for good health and wellbeing.

✤ VEGANS

If you are on a vegan or vegetarian diet, the more common deficiencies will include calcium, zinc, iron, vitamin B_{12} and protein. This is because these nutrients are more difficult to obtain in diets containing no animal products. You will need to inform yourself in detail about how to combine the different types of foods to get adequate amounts of all the building blocks of protein. Zinc is difficult to absorb because phytochemicals called phytates in grains, cereals, wholegrain breads and legumes bind zinc and stop it from being absorbed. Iron and vitamin B_{12} are difficult to maintain in adequate amounts on a vegan diet, and will often need to be supplemented, particularly in women who are menstruating.

See the following section for a list of some of the major vitamins and supplements, where they are useful, what happens when there is a deficiency, and what some of the potential adverse effects are. For information on herbs, refer to the chapter 'Herbal Medicine', on page 233.

Obviously there is not enough space in this book to include every supplement or everything you need to know about each of them, so I have listed some of the more commonly used ones, the ones that should be used more often and those that are likely to need more caution when they are taken. So, while this list isn't exhaustive, it is still extensive and not all the information may be relevant to you or your health goals. I suggest reading the first point, about what the vitamin may be prescribed for, and then deciding whether it is appropriate to you.

Vitamin A

May be prescribed for:

- *correcting deficiency – symptoms include vision problems (night blindness), thickened skin, poor dental health, impaired immunity.*

Risk of deficiency increases with coeliac disease, diseases of the pancreas, intestinal infections and infestations, diabetes, hyperthyroidism, protein deficiency.

Vitamin A is involved in maintaining healthy vision, immune function, fertility, skin function, growth and development.

Sources:

Animal products such as red meat, eggs, liver, fish and dairy products.

Interactions:

Absorption is reduced by the medications cholestyramine, orlistat and colchicine.

Statins and the oral contraceptive pill increase vitamin A levels in your blood.

Avoid taking vitamin A with the acne drug isotretinoin or the antibiotics minocycline and tetracycline.

Precautions:

Not to be taken in pregnancy or long term in high doses (over 10000 IU/day).

Toxicity:

Can be serious. Symptoms include dry skin, cracked lips, coarse hair, dry mouth, double vision, bone and joint pain, fatigue, nausea, vomiting, depression, irritability, headache, liver damage.

Vitamin B₁ (thiamine)

May be prescribed for:

- *correcting deficiency – symptoms include beriberi, fatigue, weakness, stiffness, irritability, memory loss, sleep disturbance, anorexia, constipation*
- *excessive alcohol intake*
- *anorexia*

- *times of increased need for thiamine – pregnancy, and hyperthyroidism, fever, acute infection, chronic diarrhoea, strenuous exercise, breastfeeding, and adolescent growth spurts.*

Also known as thiamine, vitamin B_1 assists your body to convert carbohydrates into energy. You need vitamin B_1 for normal brain and nerve function, and for healthy skin, eyes, hair and liver.

Very little thiamine is stored in your body, so deficiency signs can be seen within two or three weeks of restricted intake.

Food sources:

Lean meat, legumes cereals, grains, pasta, seeds, soy milk.

Deficiency causes:

In addition to the symptoms listed above, a particularly severe form of alcohol-related brain damage called Wernicke-Korsakoff syndrome is the result of thiamine deficiency and causes stumbling, poor memory and confusion.

Interactions:

Some diuretics (Lasix, frusemide), digoxin, phenytoin.

Toxicity/Overdose:

Excessive doses are eliminated in your urine so toxicity does not occur.

Vitamin B_2 (riboflavin)

May be prescribed for:

- *correcting deficiency – symptoms include fatigue, cracks in the corners of the mouth, poor wound healing, dermatitis, digestive problems, swollen red tongue, sore throat, light sensitivity, eye strain*
- *prevention of migraine headaches.*

Uses:

All B vitamins assist your body to convert carbohydrates into energy. Riboflavin also works as an antioxidant. B vitamins are usually given in combination because they work together. Riboflavin helps to convert folate and vitamin B_6 into their functional form.

Riboflavin is important for vision and the production of red blood cells.

It may reduce frequency and severity of migraine headaches.

Risk of deficiency is increased in adolescence and in the elderly, and in alcoholics.

Food sources:

Almonds, Vegemite, whole grains, wheat germ, wild rice, mushrooms, soybeans, milk, yoghurt, eggs, broccoli, Brussels sprouts, spinach.

Interactions:

Some drugs reduce your levels or interfere with the absorption of riboflavin so supplements are more likely to be needed. You will need professional advice on riboflavin supplementation if you are taking tricyclic antidepressants, antipsychotics, oral contraceptive pill, some chemotherapy drugs (doxorubicin), tetracycline, methotrexate, phenytoin, thiazide diuretics.

Precautions:

B vitamins are best taken in combination with other B vitamins.

Toxicity/Overdose:

Very high doses can cause sun damage to the eyes, and numbness, burning or prickling sensations in the skin.

Vitamin B₃ (niacin)

May be prescribed for:

- *correcting deficiency – symptoms include pellagra (cracked skin), dementia, diarrhoea (can be fatal), indigestion, fatigue, skin sores, vomiting, poor concentration, anxiety, fatigue, restlessness, apathy, depression.*

Uses:

- *all B vitamins assist your body to convert carbohydrates into energy.*

Needed for the production of sex hormones and stress-related hormones, and regulation of blood sugar levels. Decreases triglycerides and increases HDL (good cholesterol).

Sources:

Fish, sunflower seeds, peanuts. Converted from tryptophan in red meat, poultry, eggs and dairy products.

Interactions:

Interferes with tetracycline antibiotic. The epilepsy medications phenytoin and valproic acid can cause niacin deficiency.

Niacin may increase potency of blood thinning medications.

Taken with statins, niacin may improve the effectiveness of the statin but increases the risk of serious statin side effects like muscle or liver damage.

Precautions:

B vitamins are best taken in combination with other B vitamins. May affect blood sugar control in diabetes.

Toxicity/Overdose:

High doses can cause the 'niacin flush', a hot sensation with tingling and red flushed face and chest, and sometimes cause palpitations. Taking aspirin before you take niacin can prevent the flush. Very high doses can cause liver damage and stomach ulcers. May worsen gout.

Vitamin B₅ (pantothenic acid)

May be prescribed for:

- *correcting deficiency – symptoms include burning feet, gut upset and vomiting, dizziness, depression, poor immune function, fatigue, weakness.*

Uses:

All B vitamins assist your body to convert carbohydrates into energy. Vitamin B₅ reduces total cholesterol.

Deficiency is more common in people with bowel problems where absorption is reduced, alcoholics and diabetics.

Food sources:

Small amounts are found in most foods, especially meat, eggs, broad beans, legumes, whole grains, milk, avocado, mushrooms.

Interactions:

Your requirement increases if you take antibiotics or the oral contraceptive pill.

Precautions:

B vitamins are best taken in combination with other B vitamins.

Toxicity/Overdose:

Toxicity is unknown and there are no reported adverse effects.

Vitamin B₆ (pyridoxine)

May be prescribed for:

- *correcting deficiency – symptoms include dermatitis, cracked corners of the mouth, sore tongue, anaemia, impaired immunity, kidney stones, elevated homocysteine (increases heart disease risk), irritability, confusion, depression, seizures*
- *pregnancy-associated nausea*

- *premenstrual syndrome*
- *preventing progression of macular degeneration*
- *assisting symptoms of depression*
- *assisting in treatment of rheumatoid arthritis (deficiency is more common in people with rheumatoid arthritis).*

Uses:

All B vitamins assist your body to convert carbohydrates into energy. Vitamin B_6 also helps in the production of several neurotransmitters (serotonin and norepinephrine) and melatonin, and is essential for normal brain function. With vitamin B_{12} and folate, helps to control homocysteine level, associated with heart disease.

May help morning sickness, premenstrual syndrome, depression, rheumatoid arthritis and macular degeneration.

Food sources:

Fish, legumes, wheat germ, eggs, nuts, potatoes, bananas, Vegemite.

Interactions:

Some medications reduce vitamin B_6 levels. All B vitamins reduce absorption of tetracycline.

Vitamin B_6 may increase the effectiveness of tricyclic antidepressants.

B_6 may reduce the side effects of chemotherapy drugs 5-Fluorouracil and doxorubicin.

Precautions:

B vitamins are best taken in combination with other B vitamins. Taken at night, it may disrupt sleep and cause vivid dreams.

Toxicity/Overdose:

Nausea, abdominal pain, loss of appetite, sun sensitivity.

Vitamin B_{12} (cyanocobalamin)

May be prescribed for:

- *correcting deficiency – symptoms include pernicious anaemia, nerve disorder (weakness, numbness and tingling), impaired memory, irritability, depression, dementia, loss of appetite, gut disturbance.*

Uses:

- *all B vitamins assist your body to convert carbohydrates into energy.*

Sources:

Eggs, meat, dairy products, poultry, shellfish. There is no reliable vitamin B_{12} source in plant foods, so vegetarians and vegans are particularly at risk of deficiency. Deficiency is also a problem if you have absorption problems – for example, coeliac disease, Crohn's disease – and if you are aged over 50.

Interactions:

Lithium, metformin and the oral contraceptive pill decrease Vitamin B_{12} levels.

Precautions:

If absorption is a problem, vitamin B_{12} needs to be given as drops under the tongue or by regular injection.

Vitamin C

May be prescribed for:

- *correcting deficiency – symptoms include scurvy, fatigue, weakness, bruising, bleeding, poor wound healing, weight loss, irritability, depression, aches and pains, frequent infections, leg swelling, anaemia, leg pain*
- *supporting immunity*
- *reducing duration of common cold symptoms*
- *preventing heart disease*
- *adjunctive cancer treatment (megadoses given intravenously)*
- *reducing inflammation*
- *recovery from illness*
- *assisting wound healing.*

Uses:

Important in growth and healing of all body tissues, repair and maintenance of skin, blood vessels, bones and cartilage, and immune function. Helps the absorption of iron. Vitamin C is a powerful antioxidant and can help in prevention and treatment of cancer and heart disease.

Sources:

It is not possible to manufacture or store vitamin C in your body, so you need a constant regular supply. It is in many fruits and vegetables – especially citrus, blackcurrants, strawberries – but is easily destroyed by storage and cooking, and is sensitive to light.

Interactions:

Increases iron absorption and if you are iron deficient, your doctor will usually get you to take iron with vitamin C to exploit this interaction.

Toxicity/Overdose:

High oral doses can give you diarrhoea.

Vitamin D

May be prescribed for:

- *correcting deficiency – symptoms include rickets in children, osteoporosis, fatigue, increased risk of infection, weakness, increased risk of some cancers, increased severity of asthma.*

Uses:

- *vitamin D is one of the most intriguing vitamins, with many uses being discovered. It helps the body to absorb calcium and is essential for healthy bones and immune function. Adequate vitamin D is needed to reduce your risk of bowel cancer, breast cancer, heart disease, infections and autoimmune diseases. Supplements are given during pregnancy to make sure the baby has enough vitamin D for normal bone development.*

Sources:

Sun exposure is the best source, but also dairy products, fatty fish, oysters.

The 'sun safe' message has, in fact, been too successful and resulted in a virtual epidemic of vitamin D deficiency. Many people have taken the 'avoid sunburn' message to mean 'avoid sun', and are not spending enough time outdoors with their skin exposed to make the vitamin D they need to maintain healthy levels. If you are one of those people who work indoors, exercise indoors, and rarely see the outdoors for most of the week, then you are likely to be at risk of vitamin D deficiency. Just 15 minutes of sunshine on your skin without sunscreen each day (longer in the cooler months) can be enough to help your body produce adequate vitamin D. This level of exposure can be difficult or impossible to get in winter, so a supplement may be necessary to maintain your levels.

Interactions:

High doses might cause abnormal heart rhythms if you are taking digoxin.

Precautions:

You need to ask for medical advice if you have any problem with calcium levels or with your parathyroid gland, or if you have lupus or sarcoidosis and you are planning on taking high doses.

Toxicity/Overdose:

Toxicity is very uncommon. If it occurs, it might involve confusion, kidney damage, nausea, vomiting, weakness.

Vitamin E

May be prescribed for:

- *correcting deficiency – symptoms include anaemia, immune abnormalities, abnormal platelet function, liver and kidney problems, vision problems, muscle weakness*
- *preventing progression of macular degeneration, in conjunction with supplements of zinc, vitamin C and betacarotene*
- *reducing risk of heart disease, and kidney and eye problems in people with diabetes*
- *reducing pain of rheumatoid arthritis (along with standard medications).*

Uses:

Vitamin E is one of the antioxidant vitamins. It is involved in immune function, nerve function and the production of red blood cells. It can help treat period pain, premenstrual syndrome and menopause symptom, and reduce pain in arthritis.

Food sources:

Liver, cold-pressed vegetable oils, nuts, seeds, dark green leafy vegetables, avocado, sweet potato, yam, egg yolk, asparagus, soy beans, dairy products.

Interactions:

Absorption is reduced by drugs that affect fat absorption, such as orlistat and cholestyramine. Care needed with aspirin or warfarin. Interferes with absorption of beta-blockers and calcium channel blockers used to treat high blood pressure, and also tricyclic antidepressants.

Precautions:

Vitamin E may increase the risk of bleeding, so if you have impaired blood clotting, a bleeding disorder, vitamin K deficiency or if you are at risk of thrombosis or embolism, you need to ask for medical advice on dosage before you take vitamin E. Avoid high doses before surgery. Avoid taking more than 200 IU per day.

Toxicity/Overdose:

High doses can cause nausea, flatulence, diarrhoea and palpitations.

Vitamin K

May be prescribed for:

- *correcting deficiency – symptoms include impaired blood clotting, resulting in bruising and bleeding.*

Low vitamin K intake has also been associated with higher risk of osteoporosis.

Vitamin K is a fat-soluble vitamin essential for the process of blood clot formation. The two naturally occurring forms are vitamin K_1 (produced by plants) and vitamin K_2 (from animal sources and produced by intestinal bacteria).

It is also essential for bone formation.

Sources:

Green leafy vegetables and some vegetable oils (soybean, canola, and olive) are major dietary sources of vitamin K. Hydrogenation of vegetable oils can decrease the absorption and biological effect of dietary vitamin K.

Vitamin K is also produced by intestinal bacteria. Because older adults are at increased risk of osteoporosis and hip fracture, a multivitamin-mineral supplement and at least one cup of dark green leafy vegetables per day is recommended.

Interaction:

Large doses of vitamin A and vitamin E interfere with vitamin K. High doses of vitamin K might interfere with warfarin. Prolonged use of antibiotics may decrease vitamin K production by intestinal bacteria.

Toxicity:

There is no known toxicity for high doses of vitamin K_1 or vitamin K_2.

Betacarotene

May be prescribed for:

- *correcting deficiency – deficiency has been associated with breast cancer, skin cancers, rheumatoid arthritis, Alzheimer's dementia, macular degeneration and metabolic syndrome. What we don't know is whether these conditions are caused by betacarotene deficiency or whether deficiency is a result of the disease*
- *preventing progression of macular degeneration.*

Betacarotene is an antioxidant pigment, one of the group of carotenoids that give fruit and vegetables their bright red, orange or yellow colour.

Uses:

Betacarotene is converted by the body to vitamin A. It supports immunity and is important for eye health and vision. It supports healthy skin and mucous membranes. Adequate betacarotene levels protect against heart disease and cancer.

Sources:

Carrots, sweet potato, pumpkin, spinach, apricots, rockmelon, broccoli.

Interactions:

Betacarotene is a fat-soluble vitamin so it depends on fat for absorption. Drugs that reduce the absorption of fat may reduce the absorption of betacarotene from food.

Precautions:

Avoid synthetic betacarotene. If you are a smoker you are advised to avoid betacarotene supplements because there is a suggestion that it might slightly increase your risk of lung cancer.

Toxicity/Overdose:

Betacarotene is converted into vitamin A in the body but, unlike vitamin A, it is not considered toxic, even in large doses because the body only converts as much betacarotene to Vitamin A as it needs. Excessive doses can make your skin have a yellow tinge. Excessive betacarotene supplements can be dangerous to people who smoke.

Calcium

May be prescribed for:

- *improving bone strength*
- *treating osteoporosis*
- *high blood pressure*
- *reducing increased risk of colorectal cancer.*

Uses:

Calcium is necessary for the development of teeth and the development and maintenance of strong bones, and for pretty much every body function, including muscle contraction, nerve conduction, release of hormones, blood clotting, energy and immunity. Calcium might help treat premenstrual syndrome.

Sources:

Dairy, fish with soft bones.

Interactions:

If you are taking calcium and you plan to take a medication, or if you are taking a medication and you intend to take calcium, check for any specific interactions. There are quite a few special instructions for drugs and calcium. Magnesium competes with calcium and doses may need to be separated. Calcium can increase the loss of zinc in faeces and so it can contribute to zinc deficiency.

Precautions:

Get medical advice on calcium intake if you have kidney disease, heart disease or sarcoidosis.

Adverse effects:

Constipation, flatulence.

Overdose:

Nausea, vomiting, constipation, depression, lethargy.

Chromium

May be prescribed for:

- *treating insulin resistance, which can be associated with blood sugar abnormalities and obesity.*

Chromium is an essential trace mineral. Most people have less chromium in their diets than the recommended level. Deficiency is worsened by high sugar diets, steroids (which increase urine loss of chromium), overexercise, physical trauma and emotional stress.

Uses:

Supplements are used in type 2 diabetes, hypoglycaemia, being overweight and polycystic ovary syndrome.

Sources:

Wholegrain breads and cereals, eggs, cheese, bananas, spinach, mushrooms, broccoli.

Interactions:

Steroids increase urine loss of chromium. Chromium may reduce the need for blood-sugar-lowering medication. Antacids may interfere with chromium absorption. Chromium may reduce absorption of thyroid replacement medication.

Precautions:

The chromium picolinate form is preferred.

Coenzyme Q10

May be prescribed for:

- *fatigue*
- *muscle pains*
- *chronic gum disease*
- *reducing side effects of statins*
- *reducing heart damage caused by some forms of chemotherapy*
- *reducing side effects of tricyclic antidepressants*
- *increasing exercise endurance in athletes*
- *reducing blood pressure*
- *adjunctive treatment after some forms of cancer*
- *boosting immunity.*

Coenzyme Q10 is found in all cells of the body.

Uses:

Heart failure, high blood pressure, recovery from heart attack or heart surgery, angina, improving exercise tolerance, migraine, Parkinson's disease, gum disease and many others.

Sources:

Meat and oily fish, whole grains, soy, broccoli, cauliflower, spinach, nuts.

Interactions:

Coenzyme Q10 levels are reduced by statins – drugs taken to reduce cholesterol levels. May protect against the heart damage caused by some forms of chemotherapy, reduces side effects of some other drugs such as tricyclic antidepressants and statins.

Toxicity/Overdose:

No known risks.

Folate (Vitamin B$_9$)

May be prescribed for:

- *correcting deficiency – symptoms include anaemia, fatigue, irritability, depression, forgetfulness, foggy thinking, headache, hair loss, nausea, insomnia, diarrhoea, weight loss, tongue and gum inflammation*

- *reducing risk of spina bifida and other birth defects caused by folate deficiency in pregnancy.*

Folate works with vitamin B_{12} and vitamin C to help the body metabolise proteins. Folate deficiency is common. The risk of deficiency is increased by the process of cooking food, drinking alcohol and having a poor diet lacking in fresh vegetables. Food preparation and processing can destroy virtually all the folate in foods and it is sensitive to light, air and heat.

Uses:

Must be taken by all women planning pregnancy and during pregnancy to prevent brain and spinal cord defects. Helps prevent heart disease. Folate supplements help slow the progression of age-related hearing loss in elderly people with high homocysteine levels and low dietary folate.

Sources:

Spinach and other fresh green leafy vegetables, asparagus, turnip, beets, root vegetables, soybeans, salmon, avocado, milk, mushrooms, legumes, nuts, fortified cereals.

Deficiency causes:

Folic acid deficiency can result in

- *Diarrhoea*
- *Weakness*
- *Fatigue*
- *Headache*
- *Palpitations*
- *Behaviour change*
- *Irritability*
- *Grey hair*
- *Mouth ulcers*
- *Peptic ulcers*
- *Swollen tongue.*

Interactions:

Folate works with other B vitamins. There are some specific drug interactions, so check if you are taking a medication and you plan to take folate, and also check if you are taking folate and intend to take a medication. *Lots* of drugs reduce the absorption of folate, including trimethoprim, antacids, anti-epilepsy drugs, non-steroidal anti-inflammatory drugs and others.

Toxicity/Overdose:

Very high doses can cause stomach problems, sleep problems, skin reactions, seizures.

Iodine

May be prescribed for:

- *correcting deficiency, which causes hypothyroidism – symptoms include weight gain, sluggishness, dry hair and skin, intolerance to cold environment. Hypothyroidism causes mental retardation known as 'cretinism' in babies of pregnant women who are iodine deficient.*

Iodine is essential for the production of thyroid hormone. If you don't have enough iodine, you can develop goitre (thyroid gland enlargement) and underactive thyroid.

Iodine deficiency is the world's leading cause of preventable intellectual disability in children, so women who are thinking about pregnancy, or are pregnant or breastfeeding need to know their iodine status through a simple urine test. Iodine deficiency can be easily supplemented with drops.

In recent years there was a problem with a brand of soy milk that contained excessive amounts of iodine and some people who drank large quantities of the milk developed thyroid overactivity.

Uses:

Iodine is a trace mineral that the body needs to make thyroid hormone.

Sources:

Iodised salt, saltwater fish, seaweeds, dairy products.

Precautions:

Excess supplementation can cause thyroid disease.

Iron

May be prescribed for:

- *correcting deficiency, which is extremely common, especially in vegetarians and the elderly, and in women with heavy periods. Iron deficiency also occurs if you have a dietary deficiency, poor absorption, chronic illness or blood loss from bowel disease. Signs of deficiency can be subtle – tiredness, reduced exercise tolerance, increased susceptibility to infection, anaemia, breathlessness, rapid heart rate, pallor, depressed mood, intolerance to cold weather.*

If you are told you have iron deficiency, it will need to be medically investigated to identify any underlying cause.

Uses:

Iron is an essential mineral for your body functions and makes it possible for oxygen to be transported around your body.

Sources of iron

- red meat
- liver
- poultry
- oysters and shellfish
- nuts
- legumes
- egg yolk
- fruit
- dried fruit
- beetroot
- grains
- tofu

Iron absorption can be reduced by:

- *eating whole grains, spinach, chocolate, berries*
- *antacids*
- *calcium supplements and calcium-rich foods such as dairy products*
- *zinc supplements*
- *malabsorption or diarrhoea.*

Interactions:

Iron is best absorbed in the stomach and absorption is enhanced by taking it at the same time as a food or supplement containing vitamin C. Iron can interfere with the absorption of zinc and calcium so if you are taking these supplements, it should be taken at a different time.

Precautions:

Iron can cause your bowel motions to look black. It can also cause constipation. Must not be taken if you have a condition called haemochromatosis, which causes iron overload. If iron is injected intramuscularly, it can cause permanent discolouration of your skin which looks like a permanent bruise or a tattoo.

Toxicity/Overdose:

It is possible to have too much iron and there are some conditions where it is dangerous to take iron supplements. Iron overload can cause organ failure, so make sure you get medical advice before considering supplementing yourself.

Lutein and Zeaxanthin

May be prescribed for:

- *correcting deficiency, which causes increased risk of macular degeneration (a leading cause of blindness in people aged over 65).*

Uses:

- *lutein and zeaxanthin are carotenoid vitamins. High dietary intake reduces the risk of macular degeneration and cataracts, heart disease and some cancers.*

Sources:

Green leafy vegetables (kale, spinach), egg yolk, kiwifruit, grapes, zucchini, broccoli.

Interactions:

Supplements should be taken with a meal because fat improves their absorption. Activity is enhanced by vitamin C and vitamin E.

Lycopene

May be prescribed for:

- *reducing prostate cancer risk*
- *reducing heart disease risk*
- *preventing progression of macular degeneration.*

Studies of lycopene and health have referred to dietary intake, mostly of tomato-based foods, and point to lower incidence of cancer, particularly prostate cancer, heart disease and macular degeneration.

Lycopene is a bright pigment found in red fruits and vegetables that give them a yellow, red or orange colour. It is present in the blood, skin, liver, adrenal glands, lungs, colon and, in men, the prostate gland.

Uses:

Lycopene is an antioxidant.

Sources:

Tomatoes, watermelon, guava, papaya, apricots, pink grapefruit. Interestingly, lycopene availability from tomatoes in increased by cooking.

Toxicity/Overdose:

Eating very large amounts of lycopene-containing foods over a period of time can give your skin a yellowish hue. Some people might experience nausea, diarrhoea and bloating.

Magnesium

May be prescribed for:

- *correcting deficiency – symptoms include muscle cramps, muscle weakness, fatigue, twitching, constipation, irregular heartbeat, depression*
- *muscle spasm*
- *palpitations and abnormal heart rhythms*
- *fibromyalgia*
- *high blood pressure*
- *migraine headaches*
- *osteoporosis (along with calcium, vitamin D and other nutrients)*
- *premenstrual syndrome*
- *restless legs*
- *pre-eclampsia of pregnancy.*

Deficiency is very common and more so in people who drink alcohol or have poorly controlled diabetes or chronic diarrhoea. Mild magnesium deficiency might show itself as muscular tics, leg cramps, muscle weakness and tiredness. More severe magnesium deficiency can cause low calcium and potassium levels, severe muscle spasms, loss of appetite, personality changes, nausea, insulin resistance, irregular heartbeat and life-threatening heart failure.

Interactions:

A high-fat diet and some medications may decrease magnesium absorption, and cooking can decrease magnesium content in foods. Alcohol causes magnesium loss from urine. Diuretics increase urinary loss of magnesium, too. There is a complex interaction with calcium.

Sources:

Green leafy vegetables, nuts, peas, beans, legumes, wholegrain cereals.

Precautions:

Take care with doses if you have kidney problems.

Toxicity/Overdose:

Gut irritation, nausea, vomiting, diarrhoea.

Probiotics

May be prescribed for:

- *Imbalance of gut bacteria – symptoms include bloating, flatulence, abdominal pain, diarrhoea and/or constipation, fungal infection, fatigue, trouble concentrating, muscle pains, allergies.*

Your body is composed of 10 to 100 trillion cells, but these are outnumbered at least 10 times by the organisms living in your gut, the so-called gut microflora.

Uses:

A healthy balance of micro-organisms in the gut and the genital region are important in maintaining health and wellbeing. Beyond that, you can use specific types of probiotics for particular purposes or to get a particular effect.

There are two predominant types: lactobacilli and bifidobacteria. These probiotic bacteria stick to the intestinal wall, making it more difficult for the bugs that cause disease to get a hold. Lactobacilli primarily inhabit the small intestine, while bifidobacteria are found predominately in the large intestine.

Other strains are used for their therapeutic effect in conditions such as inflammatory bowel disease, diarrhoea, irritable bowel syndrome, allergies, thrush, eczema. A yeast called *saccharomyces boulardii* is commonly used to treat infectious diarrhoea, traveller's diarrhoea and as an adjunct in the treatment of some parasite infections.

Sources:

Most commonly, dairy-based yoghurt and specialised cultures are contained in specific probiotic supplements.

Interactions:

If you take antibiotics, particularly in high doses or over a long period of time, the treatment may destroy the beneficial bacteria in the gut and vagina, creating an environment that favours pathogens, the disease-causing bugs.

You will need a minimum daily oral dose of over 10 billion live organisms to effectively recolonise the intestines and vagina. It is generally recommended that you take probiotics for at least four weeks to ensure adequate recolonisation.

Precautions:

If you need to take antibiotics, probiotics need be taken twice a day, preferably with meals and at least two hours away from the antibiotic dose. If you need to take specialised probiotics, you must get professional advice.

SAMe (S-adenosyl-L-methionine)

May be prescribed for:

- *osteoarthritis (to reduce pain and inflammation)*
- *depression*
- *fibromyalgia*
- *migraine.*

SAMe has anti-inflammatory, antidepressant, pain-relieving effects and has a protective effect on the liver.

Sources:

Mainly produced in the liver. Taken as a supplement.

Interactions:

Antidepressants.

Precautions:

Avoid if you have bipolar disorder, schizophrenia or schizoaffective disorder.

Toxicity/Overdose:

Anxiety, headache, dizziness, sweating, itch.

Selenium

May be prescribed for:

- *correcting defiency, which causes poor immune function, increased risk of some cancers, poor thyroid function (especially if there is also an iodine deficiency), cardiovascular disease, asthma and rheumatoid arthritis.*

Selenium levels may be low if you smoke, drink alcohol, have a digestion problem like Crohn's disease or ulcerative colitis, or if your food supply is deficient in selenium.

Uses:

An antioxidant mineral. Plays a role in the immune system and thyroid function.

Selenium levels in food depend on the levels in the soils where the food was produced. Processing destroys selenium content.

Sources:

Whole unprocessed foods are preferable. Brazil nuts, wheat germ, liver, butter, fish and shellfish, garlic, whole grains, sunflower seeds.

Interactions:

Can increase bleeding if taken with clopidogrel, warfarin or aspirin. May interfere with chemotherapy.

Precautions:

Avoid doses over 150 mcg per day. Do not supplement if your blood levels are adequate. Ask medical advice if you have an underactive thyroid or if you are at risk of skin cancer.

Toxicity/Overdose:

Excessive doses (generally over 1000 mcg per day) can cause hair loss, muscle cramps, diarrhoea, fatigue, loss of fingernails, blistering skin, joint pain. Excessive doses (over 200 mcg per day) may increase your risk of diabetes and non-melanoma skin cancer.

Zinc

May be prescribed for:

- *correcting deficiency – deficiency causes vision and hearing loss, susceptibility to infections, hair loss, loss of taste sensation and appetite, dry skin, anaemia*
- *preventing progression of macular degeneration*
- *boosting immune system*
- *skin problems*
- *reducing symptoms of common colds*
- *reducing symptoms of cold sores*
- *acne.*

Uses:

Zinc is the key mineral for the proper functioning of the immune system and is essential for normal growth and development.

Deficiency impairs overall immune function and resistance to infection.

Zinc supplementation, especially in combination with other micro-nutrients, can enhance immunity if an underlying zinc deficiency if present.

Zinc deficiency is reasonably common because of poor absorption, low zinc content in the diet, or other factors such as age or medication.

Zinc is used topically in creams or lotions to help healing of ulcers and wounds.

Oral zinc supplements help wound healing and reduce infection.

Zinc can reduce the severity and duration of symptoms of the common cold. It is important in the diet as a trace element, as over 80 enzymes are known to require zinc for their normal activity. It has also been proposed that zinc medications may coat the common cold viruses and prevent them from attaching to the nasal cells.

Zinc can also be useful in the treatment of acne, chronic diarrhoea, anorexia nervosa, alcoholism and diabetes.

It is also used in combination with antioxidants to prevent the progression of age-related macular degeneration.

You are more likely to have a zinc deficiency if you are in one of these groups:

- *heavy drinkers (alcohol decreases zinc absorption and increases zinc loss in urine)*
- *breastfeeding mothers*
- *elderly (decreased absorption)*
- *vegetarians need 50 per cent more zinc than non-vegetarians because of lower absorption from plant foods and decreased absorption of zinc due to phytates in grain*
- *people with digestive diseases; for example, Crohn's disease and coeliac disease, as chronic diarrhoea causes zinc loss*
- *people taking acid-lowering medication or antacids, as low gastric acid lowers uptake of zinc*
- *people taking folate (may reduce zinc levels)*
- *heavy coffee drinker*
- *people prescribed blood pressure medications enalapril and captopril.*

Natural sources of dietary zinc

- ❧ oysters
- ❧ red meat
- ❧ poultry
- ❧ beans
- ❧ nuts
- ❧ some seafood
- ❧ whole grains
- ❧ dairy products

Deficiency causes:

- *recurrent infections and delayed recovery from infection*
- *delayed wound healing*
- *poor appetite and weight loss*
- *skin rashes*
- *taste and smell abnormalities*
- *retarded growth and development in children*
- *hair loss*
- *low sperm count in men*
- *diarrhoea*
- *mental lethargy.*

Interactions:

The diuretic amiloride reduces zinc excretion and can lead to excess zinc levels. If taking zinc supplements and a non-steroidal anti-inflammatory drug, separate the doses by at least two hours.

Precautions:

In high doses zinc can cause nausea, vomiting and gastric upset.

Toxicity/Overdose:

Overdosage can cause altered iron function, anaemia, reduced immune function (leukopenia or low white blood cells), diarrhoea, nausea and vomiting.

Zinc is toxic if taken in high doses over long periods of time. It can also cause low copper levels and interfere with iron absorption.

What you need to know:

Have your zinc level checked with a zinc taste test. Since zinc is so intimately associated with the taste function, researchers led by

Dr Derrick Bryce-Smith at Reading University in England discovered that a specially prepared solution of zinc, when taken orally, could be used to determine zinc status. In their studies (published in the *Lancet* in 1985) they found that after 10 ml of the oral Zinc Taste Test solution was held in the mouth, a lack of taste or a delayed taste perception indicated a zinc deficiency state. An immediate taste perception of the solution suggests that your zinc levels are adequate.

Assess your diet and ensure you have adequate zinc in your food.

Consider added zinc if you are deficient in zinc, if you are in a risk group, and during the treatment of acute infections and skin conditions.

MOVING FORWARD

YOUR GOALS

Goal	Activity	Obstacles/solutions	Result
Target vitamin D deficiency	Go for a walk outside for 15 minutes per day	Making the time: plan to do the walk every day	Deficiency is corrected

HEALTH AND SAFETY WARNINGS

When you are managing your own health, bear in mind that there are some pitfalls to consider with drugs, herbs, vitamins and nutritional supplements.

- *Many information sources are inaccurate or misleading.*

- ***There is potential for interactions*** *between prescriptions, medicines/ herbs/supplements, or alcohol and other drugs or treatments, which may not be advised on the label.*

- ***You need to be on the alert for risky combinations****; for example, between St John's wort and common prescription antidepressants.*

- *Detailed credible information about a therapeutic substance is often not provided, not understood, or may not be in your first language. Some medicines information has little advice on safety in pregnancy or for use in children.*

- ***Do not stop taking essential prescribed medication*** *or reduce or alter your dosages without medical advice.*

- *If you have been prescribed nutritional supplements or herbal remedies, make sure you have a timeframe for how long you are expected to take it before you see an improvement, and make a time for a follow-up visit to review the action plan rather than continuing to buy the same supplements without review.*

- ***Beware internet purchases****. Are you taking what you think you are taking? Internet suppliers are notoriously unreliable. Some websites operate legally and within appropriate safeguards for the products they sell and protect your privacy, but others are downright shonky, without safeguards for the quality of their products. The website might look legitimate but it can be a front for an illegal supplier with drugs containing the wrong type or amount of the active ingredient, or no active ingredient, or a drug that may contain dangerous additives. The safest way to obtain pharmaceuticals is through a community pharmacist. Herbal and vitamin supplements vary widely in their quality, and the most reliable suppliers will have high quality products with professional advice available at the dispensary. If you decide to buy drugs or supplements over the internet, it is very difficult to tell which websites are legitimate suppliers. A legitimate supplier should require a medical or registered professional prescription for your order, it will be located in your country, and there should be a contact number that answers with a* *real person when you call to check, and a means of protecting your private medical information. A registered pharmacist should be available to answer any queries you have. If the prices are dramatically lower than the competition, then be very cautious. There may be a reason for the price cut, but it is unlikely to be a good one.*

Step 3

SUSTAIN

Your New Normal

Final Thoughts

Your New Normal

By now you have audited your life and lifestyle and worked out the areas where you need to make changes. More importantly, you have decided what you are prepared to change, you have rebooted your lifestyle and you are ready for the next step. You can now set your long-term goals and put a plan in place to achieve these goals.

> LET'S CALL IT YOUR NEW NORMAL. Your new healthier lifestyle will become your new normal way of living.

If you have ever moved to a new country, a different city or even just moved house, you will know that it takes a while to develop new patterns and for those patterns to start to feel 'normal'. After a few weeks or months of living in a new house, you get that feeling of coming home and feeling like you are 'at home'. After you have undergone any significant shift in the way you live there will be a similar phase of adjustment. The challenge is to hold onto the new patterns that you know are in the best interest of your plan for ultimate wellness until they feel like second nature, especially if they feel uncomfortable or alien at first.

Some people I work with on their wellness program feel so invigorated and energised after just a short time that they have no problem keeping up the new pattern. But it is not always so easy or straightforward. Often I speak to people who have taken on a fad diet and can't wait to get back to their old favourite foods. And there are the people who go to a health resort and eat salads, exercise, and do yoga and meditation every day for a couple of weeks but let it all go the minute they drive past a fast food outlet on their way home. Some people really struggle with the withdrawal from drugs or cigarettes and wonder if it is worth it.

Your reboot phase is your opportunity to look with fresh eyes at the health decisions you make every hour of every day. This next phase is to work out which changes you need to sustain, and to establish your new healthy lifestyle as your permanent lifestyle.

Ultimate wellness is about deciding you want to live the healthiest life you can from now on, without feeling as if you are making a gigantic, unsustainable sacrifice. You must make a clear distinction in your mind that 'getting healthy' is not a project or a fad. It is not a punishment or a way of atoning for past sins. Rather, it is a willing transition to a permanent change to your life and lifestyle.

Whether your reboot has been a few minor adjustments or a drastic upheaval of everything you think and do, it is an opportunity to look at how you want to live your life, being mindful of the trade-offs between your decisions and behaviours and the consequences for your health. I have spoken about mindfulness a number of times and it's something you can practice every hour of every day. The choices you make affect your ability to achieve ultimate wellness. And those choices belong solely to you.

So now comes the next challenge. Step three is sustain.

WHAT DOES YOUR NEW NORMAL LOOK LIKE?

Go back to your Health Audit (on page 15) and see where you began. Then look at the changes you decided to make as a part of your rebooting process. Maybe you decided on a total detox of yourself, your home and your workplace. Or perhaps you decided on some less ambitious, incremental changes in some areas of your lifestyle.

Once you have achieved your short-term reboot goals, it is time to set up a picture of your new normal. This will be a careful assessment of what you can realistically expect to integrate into your life on a permanent basis, or at least for the foreseeable future. If it doesn't feel like second nature at first, with time and persistence it will.

TRANSITIONING YOUR NEW HEALTHY LIFESTYLE INTO YOUR NEW NORMAL

On the way to transitioning your healthy lifestyle to your new normal lifestyle, you'll need to find the impetus to put into place your new way of living and to keep it going.

Motivation is a big factor. If you find you feel instantly better after you make a change, then you will have the ready-made motivation to keep doing what you are doing. For example, let's say as part of your detox you stopped drinking alcohol and discovered you really feel a lot better for it. You might decide that you will not start drinking alcohol again, but if you do, your plan will be to stay within the safe levels and not binge drink any more.

YOUR LONG-RANGE SUSTAIN PLAN

This is your wish list for your plan for ultimate wellness. Think about what you want to achieve and what ongoing action you will take to achieve it. List any barriers or obstructions you come across and then, using the information you have gained, think about possible ways around those barriers or obstructions. Ask yourself these questions:

- *What are my health priorities?*
- *What can I change?*
- *What am I prepared to change now?*
- *What am I prepared to change down the track?*
- *How committed am I to the change?*
- *What are the likely or real obstacles and what are the practical ways to get around them? (See the next section for some help with this.)*

TROUBLESHOOTING

Change does not always go smoothly. If you hit a bump, that's when you need to move into troubleshooting mode. Let's look at some of the barriers and obstacles that commonly come up and ways to get around them.

DETOURS

There are some people who find the transition to their new normal is an easy one-way trip. Then there's everyone else. There are the patients who tell me they have 'failed' because they quit smoking for a while and restarted, or they started an exercise program and stopped because they got busy at work or had an injury.

If you keep your mind on the goal of ultimate wellness, then you have not failed. Look at the reasons you went off track rather than seeing your attempt as a failure. These experiences teach you about yourself and what will and won't work for you. These are the times to go back to your Health Audit, reset your short-term goals in the areas where you are having difficulty and start over.

> The road to ultimate wellness can have bends and detours, the occasional red light and wrong turn.

'I DON'T FEEL BETTER YET'

One of the first obstacles is delayed gratification. If you are expecting instant results, or to see results within a few days or weeks, then you may be disappointed that you are not feeling better yet.

I acknowledge it is difficult when you have made the hard changes and you do not feel instantly better. Or you actually feel worse initially. I sometimes see this with smokers, at least for a while. Some people who quit smoking really miss the camaraderie of the smoko, some suffer withdrawal effects and others miss the pleasure surge they used to get from nicotine ... the short-term reinforcement of an unhealthy habit. This can also happen with withdrawal from addictive substances like alcohol, caffeine and other drugs.

In this situation, in order to get past the early difficulties, you need to be utterly convinced that you are making an effective long-term investment in your health. It's like buying shares in a company and then having to wait years to see a return on your investment. You might have to make a leap of faith to believe that the short-term discomfort will be worth the eventual wellness.

Think about the reasons you decided to make the change in the first place. Was it because you have been diagnosed with a disease? Your children are worried about you? Your relationship is in trouble? You feel tired, stressed or miserable most of the time?

Remind yourself of those reasons. If the 'boots and all' approach is too much for you initially, pick the most important and achievable intervention. You may need help from your doctor to decide the top priority. Stick with that before you move onto lower order issues.

Impatience can be a problem, too. Don't give up because you wanted to feel different quickly. Consider the timeframes. If your unhealthy habits have gone on for a long time, then the timeframe to feel a difference might also be longer.

EXCUSES VERSUS REASONS

Ultimate wellness is about taking responsibility for yourself and your health. In order to achieve a long-term change, you will have to do just that: change. It is worth considering what might hold you back from making the permanent changes you need to make.

Are your reasons real barriers? If it's a genuine problem, you need to be prepared to see the answer and implement practical solutions to overcome these barriers. For instance, having a new baby makes it difficult to get out to exercise every day. I remember after my first baby was born and I wanted to get back into shape. Jogging prams had not been invented then but I would put her in the regular pram and off we would go for a brisk walk every day.

If you think you can't keep up your healthy eating plan because you travel a lot, think about packing food for short trips, or organising special meals ahead with your accommodation. For longer stays, you might be able to find a hotel room with a small kitchen and refrigerator and on your arrival make a trip to the nearest supermarket for fresh ingredients. There is a way around almost every barrier.

Or are your reasons really just excuses and deep down you don't truly want to change, or don't want it enough? If this is the case, go back to your Health Audit and reconsider your health priorities. If you are not ready to change, nothing is going to happen.

> Whatever the obstacles to ultimate wellness, there is a strategy to help you overcome them.

FINDING THE TIME

'I just don't have time.' Is that a reason or an excuse? We all have busy lives with a lots of different commitments. You need to carve out time for yourself to do the things that will keep you well. Take a moment to assess where you can carve out your time and plan ahead and commit to it. For example, are you able to negotiate flexible hours with work so you can exercise more, or attend physiotherapy or dental appointments or whatever it is you need to do?

If you are finding it difficult to make time to get to the supermarket, look for a website that delivers groceries. Can you negotiate with your partner around your kids' activities to open up a bit more time for yourself? Could you reduce the time you spend on social media or watching television and use some of that time to pursue your health goals? Or can you make better use of your time – for example, could you schedule a walking meeting with a client instead of sitting down for a coffee? Can you keep your gym gear or a pair of walking shoes at work and use your lunchbreak to get some exercise?

Check your diary and delete the events or meetings that are not high priority, or cause you great stress with little return for your efforts.

It's not easy to make time for yourself but if you are serious about improving your health, you need to schedule it into your diary just as you would an important meeting.

'I'M TOO BUSY LOOKING AFTER OTHERS – I CAN'T THINK ABOUT MYSELF'

I see a lot of people in my practice who are caring for either an elderly parent, a disabled family member, young children or a sick friend. Carers often put their own health and wellbeing last. Someone recently told me that they always found the airplane safety message of 'put your oxygen mask on first, then assist children' to be confusing and counterintuitive. Until they realised that if you don't have your oxygen mask on first, you won't *be able* to help your children. This metaphor rings true for your health in general. If you don't have your wellbeing (your 'oxygen') up to scratch first, you won't have the personal resources to help the others who are depending on you. So if you are a carer, of any kind, be sure to reserve some time and energy for your own health care.

FLUSHING OUT SABOTEURS

Saboteurs come in all shapes and sizes, and they have lots of different motivations. Saboteurs are the people who, for reasons of their own, don't want you to change. Maybe your best friend likes the fact that you are both overweight, because she is not ready to change and does not want you to be slimmer than she is.

I remember the story about a husband and wife who were both clinically obese. The wife really wanted to lose weight and started out with good intentions. She cleared the fridge and pantry of all her 'naughty foods' and paid close attention to her eating plan. She would start to see results, but then would gradually put the weight back on. It turned out that her husband would come home from work with a litre of gourmet ice-cream and a box of her favourite chocolates. After dinner he would go to the fridge and serve out two bowls of ice-cream, even though she said she didn't want it. Once it was in front of her, the temptation often proved too great. Her husband did not want to change his lifestyle, and her new pattern felt like a threat to him. Eventually they agreed to disagree by talking about her desire to lose weight without him feeling pressure to do the same until he was ready.

Sometimes saboteurs have very benign motives, such as the 'feeders' who believe they are looking after you if they feed you all the food they know you love – and lots of it. These people gain pleasure from feeling they are nurturing others. When rejecting their food, explain that you are not rejecting them. Explain that looking after you means helping you to achieve your health goals. You will need to have a clear idea of the types and quantities of food you want in your diet and select them out of the food offered to you to regain control.

Maybe it is your partner who likes to have a cigarette with you and doesn't like it that you don't want to be her smoking buddy. She keeps offering you cigarettes, saying, 'What harm can just one cigarette do?' The other possible motive is that the saboteur feels guilty that they still smoke or have other unhealthy habits. What does your decision to change mean about their decision not to?

Identifying the saboteurs and their methods will help you recognise what is happening. It may be effective to speak to your saboteurs to explain that you have made decisions about your health and that you want to give it your best shot, and that you would very much appreciate their support with it. If they do not want to respect your wishes, then you will need to limit the time you spend with them, or just decide not to discuss it with them but get on with your plan quietly and deliberately.

Any element of wellness can be vulnerable to a saboteur. If there is a relationship rift in your life that is causing you distress, you might decide you are going to try to heal it. A saboteur might decide that doesn't suit them. Your attempt to change the dynamic within a family or friendship group might upset their perceived position or power structure within that group. Whether you will be successful or not will depend on how important it is to *both* you and the other person to heal the rift. This is the sort of situation that might benefit from the help of a professional counsellor.

'CATCH THE CONTAGION OF HEALTH'

One of the reasons you might go back to unhealthy habits is if you are in a relationship or a friendship group with people who don't share your newfound enthusiasm for being healthy. After studying the social connections and body composition of nearly 12,000 people participating in the Framingham Heart Study over three decades, Harvard researchers concluded that obesity was 'contagious'.

They found that clusters of obese people extended through social networks to three degrees of separation. A person's chances of becoming obese increased by 57 per cent if they had a friend who became obese. Friends of the same sex had more influence on this effect than friends of the opposite sex. If one spouse became obese, the likelihood that the other spouse would become obese increased by 37 per cent. Having four obese friends doubled a person's chance of becoming obese compared to people with no obese friends.

The researchers suggested a number of reasons for this observation, including an altered view about the acceptability of being overweight as 'normal', and copying of other people's behaviours. For example, it is hard for a new non-smoker to go out with a group of smokers and resist the temptation to light up 'just this once'.

In general practice we are usually the first to see contagions of infective diseases like influenza or gastroenteritis. We are also the first to see 'contagions' of healthy lifestyle in groups of friends where one is diagnosed with a serious medical condition and the others, knowing they have had a lucky escape so far, decide to cut their losses and get with the program.

Some years ago I noticed a sudden influx of men in their fifties, all working in the same area of business, turning up asking for heart health checks. Of course I did a comprehensive general men's health check, which included heart disease risk factors. I asked, as I often do, about the motivation for this particular health check-up. It turned out that this was a group of colleagues who had always partied hard. A few weeks before, one of them had suffered a heart attack. Visiting him in the coronary care unit, his mates had decided en masse that the time had come to reassess their lifestyle. Interestingly, years later none of this particular group had taken up smoking again and they were all watching their diet and getting regular exercise. If the people around you have the lifestyle that will keep you healthy, that will help you to keep on track.

You may need to change your social environment until you are strong enough to resist temptation. This might mean spending more time with people with the lifestyle you want to adopt in the long term. At the very least, spend the most time with people who are supportive of you and your goals. You might find these people in your extended family or broader friendship group. You might have to join groups like a gym, walking club, or tennis or walking group. It is also in your interest to recruit the people around you to audit and reboot their lifestyle, too. That way you can reinforce each other's resolve. You never know. You may become their inspiration for change.

If your partner or family members do not want to go on the program with you, then talk to them about how they can support your efforts, or at least avoid undermining you.

TALK TO YOUR OLDER SELF

Psychologists have a technique of asking you to speak to yourself as a child. I have often seen articles or blogs asking the question 'What would you say to your sixteen-year-old self?' But I am going to ask you to do something more challenging. I am asking you to speak to your *older* self. Think of yourself ten or twenty years older. Speak to the you that has benefitted from the changes you have decided to make in your life and know that your older self will be better off for the care you are taking from now on. Then consider your older self if you do not sustain these changes. How will you justify the heart attack or the stroke that could have been avoided if you had given up smoking? How will you explain that you can't take that overseas trip because your health won't allow it? Think about your responsibility to your older self. You will find this will boost your motivation. Your older self can be the beneficiary in a decade or two or more of your new normal.

RESISTING TEMPTATION

Realistically, you won't be able to eliminate all the saboteurs and obstacles from your life. This is why you will need to develop day to day, hour to hour and even moment to moment resistance strategies so that in any environment you can withstand peer pressure or temptation by keeping your eye on the prize: ultimate wellness. Here are some ideas on how to resist temptation.

❧ REMIND YOURSELF

If you are tempted to stray from your plan in the early stages of your new lifestyle, start by reminding yourself of your goals. Why am I making changes? Look at the work you have done to get this far and make the decision not to turn back.

❧ SAY 'NO' NICELY

There is a hilarious scene in one of my favourite Monty Python movies, *The Meaning of Life*, where a grossly overweight man tells the waiter that if he eats one more thing he will explode. The waiter persists in trying to get him to eat more: 'It's just wafer thin, sir.' The man relents and, literally, explodes.

> If you mean 'no', you have to say it. And if you say 'no', you have to mean it.

You might need to practise saying 'no' in a variety of ways so that people around you understand that pressuring you is not doing you any favours.

❧ THINK 'MAYBE LATER'

If you are tempted by food that you know you will later regret eating, think to yourself, 'Not now, maybe later.' Postponing the instant fulfilment of your temptation to eat something you know you shouldn't will reduce the chance that you will actually eat it. Telling yourself that you have the option to eat it later will help you to overcome the feeling of forced restraint and reinforce the fact that you are the one making a healthy choice.

Friday night – all bets are off!

In our family, on Friday nights we treat ourselves to some tasty and not always super-healthy food at the end of a long week. As part of your new normal, you need to have balance, so pick one day where you can eat a little of whatever you want, within reason and without being excessive, so your new healthy lifestyle doesn't become a repressive regime. You don't have to miss out – you just have to keep the balance.

❧ A LITTLE CAN GO A LONG WAY

When I am talking to people about their reboot process, there is often a moment of anticipatory grief that they will have to give up their great love in life, whether that is chocolate or coffee or a glass of wine. As the old saying goes, absence really can make the heart grow fonder. Rather than thinking you have to 'give up everything', think about the changes as finding a new level. Instead of four or five coffees a day, cut back to one or two and have it with skim rather than full cream milk. Have a square or two of dark chocolate instead of half a bar of milk chocolate. Drink alcohol in moderation, at safe levels. You get the picture. A little of a good thing can go a long way.

WHAT TO DO IF YOU FALL OFF THE WAGON

Once your sustain plan is in place, you might find there are times when you fall off the wagon. This can happen to anyone, particularly at times of stress. For example, you have a pressing deadline at work and you have trouble finding the time to exercise for a week or two. You go on holidays or the temptations of party season take you off target. You might face a family crisis with a sick child or parent. But rather than having your new routine fall to pieces, there are a couple of strategies you can use.

REVISIT YOUR MOTIVATION

Remind yourself of the reason you started reading this book. What was it about your life that you felt needed changing so that you could achieve ultimate wellness? Use that thought as your motivator to get yourself going again. If you've hit an obstacle and your routine has broken down, that's not the end. Just get back up and on it again.

PLAN AHEAD

If you have a busy time coming up at work, think about your exercise opportunities. Take the stairs instead of the lift, walk part of the way to work, take your walking shoes with you to the office and go for a couple of 20-minute walks during the day, even while you make important calls on your mobile phone.

Even while you are travelling or if there is a big change in your schedule, you can maintain the principles of your healthy lifestyle if you are organised.

DO A 'MINI-REBOOT'

If you do go off track a bit, it is time for a 'mini-reboot'. This is where you recognise after a week or two that you are not keeping to your lifestyle plan and you go back to your Health Audit. Look at your current practices and see where you are having trouble. Spend some time planning a strategy to overcome the barriers you are facing and putting new solutions in place.

WERE YOUR CHANGES TOO BIG?

There is a possibility your original plan may have been too ambitious at that particular time in your life. One of the secrets to success in the sustain stage is to be honest with yourself about how realistic your goals are. See small improvements as steps on the road to success.

There is no need to set yourself a difficult goal like finishing the New York marathon. If that's not on your bucket list, leave it to the marathon runners. If walking for 45 minutes a day and starting a resistance training program is achievable, then that is a realistic goal.

Weight loss goals are another area where common sense needs to prevail. If you try to lose weight too quickly and you hate the process, then as soon as you get bored with it or you feel starved and irritable, you will go back to your old comfortable overeating patterns.

The eating plan – notice I didn't say diet – you choose to make your new normal has to be something you feel happy to maintain, but which fulfils the principles of balanced nutrition and maintaining a healthy weight. So if you fall off the wagon because your changes were too ambitious, go back to your goal setting and set the bar at a realistic, maintainable level. You may need to see a dietician to work through the elements of your eating plan and see that you are getting all of the necessary nutrients and to work with your food preferences to keep you on track.

One thing I learnt from watching the Paralympics in 2012 is that for almost every obstacle, there is a solution. Rather than thinking about all the excuses of why you have to procrastinate or avoid change, think of all the reasons you want to live a more vibrant life.

I will start you off with some suggestions, and then you can individualise your plan using the information in the book, and with input from your health advisers.

YOUR LONG-RANGE PLAN

Goal	Action	Barriers and obstacles	Solutions	Result

FINAL THOUGHTS

MY JOURNEY: PART TWO

Back in 2003, when I was lying in that hospital bed during the most terrifying health crisis of my life, it took a while for the reality of the situation to sink in. Although I realised on an intellectual level that I was lucky to have survived, on an emotional level I was angry that it had happened and frightened of the long-term consequences.

My greatest fear was that I would have permanent damage as a result. It took me a while to understand that my life was about to change. That it *had* to change. Not just in the days and weeks ahead, but forever.

The day after my embolism, I was still in the intensive care unit and I tried to negotiate with the attending physician to be released over the weekend so I could go to a doctors' political rally! He told me quite firmly that I wouldn't be going anywhere. He was quite right of course. Clearly reality had not yet set in for me.

There were so many things running through my head as I lay there in that bed: you have a lot of time to think when you are lying in hospital! I thought about how I'd always been so fit and mindful of a healthy life-style. I'd been an aerobics instructor for heaven's sake! And yet, here I was. An attempted 'quick fix' hormone treatment had resulted in a threat to my life. It was true, I knew, that in the past couple of frantically busy years things had slipped a bit. And if I was really honest with myself, I knew that I had been subconsciously putting my wellbeing on the backburner. I could have made time in my schedule to exercise more, but I didn't. I could have modified my schedule, but I felt that the seriousness of the medico-political issues I was dealing with demanded long hours and constant vigilance.

After the acute crisis, I knew I would get better. The question was: how much better?

A few days after the embolism, I could just make it to the toilet ensuite in my room and back, and I'd be breathless. I thought to myself, *Is this as good as it's going to get? This can't be how my life will be.* A possible consequence of my condition was a strain on the heart that would limit my ability to do anything that required physical exertion. I couldn't face the possibility that I wouldn't be able to do the physical activities I liked ever again. I realised that I had been taking my previous good health for granted. By day eight,

I could with assistance walk across the road. I was anxious about walking more than a short distance. The embolism had shattered my confidence. When I left hospital, I had a plan to start building up my walking, bit by bit. I would start with two 10-minute walks a day. It wasn't much, but that's all I could manage to do. Over the next few weeks I built up to two 45-minute walks a day. Gradually my fitness did improve.

After a month I was back at work. Two months later I gave my final televised speech as President of the Australian Medical Association at the National Press Club in Canberra. Looking back on the recording of that one-hour speech, I can see that I was breathless towards the end.

My improvement then plateaued. I was good enough to get around but I knew I was under par. I wasn't *nearly* as fit and healthy as I had been or believed I could be. I wondered if I'd ever get that back.

I was convinced I was going to be permanently ill. I thought I would never be able to ski again and I grieved for the loss of my physical abilities. As tough as it was, deep down, I never really gave up. I gradually challenged myself with harder exercise. I saw a variety of practitioners to assist me with opening my chest movements to help me breathe differently.

I took up kayaking to exercise my upper body. I took on a trainer who pushed me enough but was also supportive and knew when not to push me too hard.

I took advice about supplements to help my exercise tolerance and energy levels.

Oh so gradually, I improved. For my fiftieth birthday my wife Jackie said, 'We're going to Aspen for you to ski.' I was anxious. I wasn't sure I could exercise at altitude. But when I went up in that chair lift, stepped off at the top and began to ski down the mountain, I experienced one of the most exhilarating moments of liberation I've ever felt in my life. In that moment, I knew I'd be okay. That was seven years after the embolism. I will never take wellbeing for granted again.

YOUR JOURNEY

You began this journey towards ultimate wellness for a reason. You were not happy or satisfied with aspects of your wellbeing, and you sensed that it was within your power to do something to change that.

In auditing your life and your lifestyle, you discovered the things you needed to do if you were going to achieve your goal of ultimate wellness.

You then faced decisions about what you were prepared to do. You put the elements of your personal plan together and got underway with the changes.

Looking to the future, your challenge is to sustain your progress. Especially when the going gets tough. At times progress will seem slow and you may question the value of the changes you are making. Remind yourself that it will be worth the effort.

The influences on your health and wellbeing go back to factors that were present before your conception, so that even with the healthiest possible lifestyle, it is not possible to be immune to health problems forever. But by living the best you can, you improve your chances of surviving health challenges and achieving ultimate wellness. You can change your life and your lifestyle for the better. You can sustain these changes. Remember to make the most of the abilities that you have. You don't have to run the New York marathon. Ultimate wellness is about getting to your 100, reaching your individual potential.

The investment you are making in your health is not just for today and tomorrow it is for 10, 20, 30, years ahead. The way you choose to live is as an investment in your long-term wellbeing. It's a positive lifestyle decision. Don't wait for a crisis to reconsider. Do it today. Whatever your motivation, the point that is a bit of effort is all it takes to get you there.

Committing to your wellbeing and setting your sights on the goal of ultimate wellbeing is the best investment you can make for your future.

Welcome to your new normal.

ACKNOWLEDGEMENTS

The research for this book took more than thirty years. Honestly! Since I started medical school, I embarked on a lifelong journey of learning about health and wellbeing, all that time evolving my approach and discovering not just the facts and statistics about disease and its medical treatment, but the philosophies and techniques of patient care and health promotion.

Over that time I have been inspired to find answers by the courage and vitality of people facing major life and health challenges with optimism and determination. They have driven me to try harder and do more to help them on their quest for ultimate wellbeing. This book owes much to those patients.

Over the course of my career I have also been inspired by colleagues who have encouraged me to think tangentially. My brother-in-law Prof Phillip Stricker is one of a rare species: an integrative surgeon who encouraged me think about how to incorporate natural therapies and lifestyle modification into the management of patients with prostate cancer before anyone else I knew was even aware of their potential in the practice of oncological surgery.

Thank you to my colleagues and staff at uclinic and Cooper Street Clinic for your professional support and for contributing to the environment of clinical excellence we have created together.

I would particularly like to acknowledge some of the clinical and academic leaders in the integrative medicine field in Australia: Dr Craig Hassed, Dr Vicki Kotsirilos, Prof Marc Cohen, Dr Lily Tomas and Dr Lesley Braun and many others who have contributed so much to the evolution of integrative medicine as the 'emerging mainstream'.

Thank you especially to Samantha Sainsbury and Ingrid Ohlsson at Pan Macmillan for their constructive and creative input into the development of the book. Thanks also to Glenda Downing, Emma Louise Gough and Jo Lyons.

Finally, huge thanks to my wife Jackie who is my constant source of emotional support and intellectual provocation, and who managed to keep our lives flowing along a smoothly as possible so I was able to immerse myself in this project.

NOTES

Page

7. '*A broad domain of healing resources …*': LS Wieland et al., Mar–Apr 2011, 'Development and classification of an operational definition of complementary and alternative medicine for the Cochrane Collaboration Altern Ther Health Med', 17(2): 50–59, viewed 16 October 2012, http://www.ncbi.nlm.nih.gov

8. '*Integrative medicine (IM) is the practice of …*': Consortium of Academic Health Centers for Integrative Medicine, 25 May 2012, Minneapolis, USA, www.imconsortium.org

9. 'Complex group of reading, listening …': US Department of Health and Human Services, 1 February 2012, Healthy People, 2012, US Federal Government, http://www.healthypeople.gov/2020

STEP 2: REBOOT
SECTION 1 CHOOSING THE RIGHT HEALTH PROFESSIONALS

Page

39. An interesting survey of Australian GPs in 2005 …: MM Cohen et al., 'The Integration of Complementary Therapies in Australian General Practice: Results of a National Survey', *The Journal of Alternative and Complementary Medicine*, vol.11, no.6, 2005, pp. 995–1104.

SECTION 2 DETOX

Page

54. *The* Journal of the American Medical Association *published an opinion that* …: DL Davis, GE Dinse, DG Hoel, 'Decreasing cardiovascular disease and increasing cancer among whites in the United States from 1973 through 1987', *JAMA*, vol. 271, 1994, pp. 431–437.

54. *The* British Medical Journal *agreed* …: RM Sharpe and SD Irvine,

'How strong is the evidence of a link between environmental chemicals and adverse effects on human reproductive health?' *British Medical Journal*, vol. 328, 2004, pp. 447–451.

57.   Exposure to VOCs can cause ...: United States Environmental Protection Agency, 09 July 2012, 'An Introduction to Indoor Air Quality. Volatile Organic Compounds', http://www.epa.gov/iaq/voc.html

SECTION 3 REBOOT YOUR LIFESTYLE

🍃 CHAPTER 2: ALCOHOL

Page

67.   The current recommendation is for ...: Department of Health and Aging, April 2012, 'Reduce Your Risk: new national guidelines for alcohol consumption', Australian Government, viewed 20 October 2012, http://www.alcohol.gov.au/internet/alcohol/publishing.nsf/Content/guide-adult

68.   Despite the fact that alcohol ...: Preventive Health Taskforce, June 2009, 'Technical Paper 3: Preventing Alcohol-related harm in Australia: a window of opportunity', Commonwealth of Australia, viewed 20 October 2012, www.health.gov.au

69.   Death from acute alcohol ...: ibid.

69.   Alcohol use disorder is ...: ibid.

69.   During the 10 years from 1993 to 2002 ...: T Chikritzhs, R Pascal and P Jones, November 2004, 'Under-aged Drinking Among 14–17 year olds and Related Harms in Australia', *National Alcohol Indicators*, Bulletin 7, Australian Government Department of Health and Ageing, http://ndri.curtin.edu.au/local/docs/pdf/naip/naip007.pdf

72.   Approximately 40 per cent of Australian men ...: CE Coulson, et al., 'Patterns of alcohol use and associated physical and lifestyle characteristics according to new Australian guidelines', *Australian and New Zealand Journal of Psychiatry*, 2010; 44: pp. 946–951.

73.   Recently we have recognised ...: Cancer Council Australia, June 2011, 'Position Statement Alcohol and Cancer Risk', http://www.cancer.org.au

73.   A recent international study ...: K Graham et al., 'Alcohol-related negative consequences among drinkers around the world', *Addiction* vol. 106, Issue 8, August 2011, pp. 1391–1405.

Page

79.   Smoking kills more men than women ...: Cancer Council NSW, 'Statistics on Smoking in Australia', viewed 21 October 2012, http://www.cancercouncil.com.au

79.   In Australia, greater awareness ...: ibid.

79.   In 1945, at the end ...: ibid.

79.   By comparison, the number ...: ibid.

79.   Although the death rates ...: ibid.

79.   In 2004, 18 per cent ...: ibid.

79.   Adolescent girls who smoke ...: I Sorheim, A Johannessen, A Gulsvik, P Bakke, E Silverman, D DeMeo, 2010, 'Chronic obstructive pulmonary disease: Gender differences in COPD: are women more susceptible to smoking effects than men?', *Thorax*, 2010; 65: pp. 480–485· doi:10.1136/thx.2009.122002, viewed 21 October 2012, http://thorax.bmj.com

79.   Women aged 45 to 74 ...: D Gold and X Wang, 'Effects of cigarette smoking on lung function in adolescent boys and girls', *New England Journal of Medicine*, 26 September 1996; 335(13): pp. 931–7.

79.   Because the lethal poisons from ...: National Cancer Institute, 'Women and Smoking', National Institute of Health, http://www.cancer.gov/cancertopics/factsheet/Tobacco/women

80.   Women who smoke have ...: I Sorheim, A Johannessen, A Gulsvik, P Bakke, E Silverman, D DeMeo, 'Chronic obstructive pulmonary disease: Gender differences in COPD: are women more susceptible to smoking effects than men?'

80.   Smokers are younger ...: ibid.

80.   In pregnant women ...: B Magee and D Hattis, 'Role of smoking in low birth weight', *The Journal of Reproductive Medicine*, January 2004; 49 (1): pp. 23–7.

80.   While you might think ...: NSW Government, 3 October 2007, 'Smoking and Pregnancy', http://www0.health.nsw.gov.au/factsheets/general/smoking_preg.html

80.   If a mother smokes ...: M McDonnell-Naughton and C McGarvey, 'Maternal smoking and alcohol consumption during pregnancy as risk factors for sudden infant death', *Irish Medical Journal*, April 2012; 105 (4): pp. 105–8.

82. One study of US college students ...: S Moran et al., 2004, 'Social Smoking Among US College Students', *Pediatrics*, http://pediatrics. aappublications.org/content/114/4/1028.abstract

86. One US study published ...: H Alpert et al., 'A prospective cohort study challenging the effectiveness of population-based medical intervention for smoking cessation Tobacco Control', *Tobacco Control*, 12 November 2012, doi:10.1136/tobaccocontrol-2011–050129

89. According to the American Cancer Society ...: American Cancer Society, 1 Feb 2012, 'When Smokers Quit What Is The Benefit Over Time?', http://www.cancer.org/healthy/stayawayfromtobacco/ guidetoquittingsmoking/guide-to-quittingsmoking-benefits

❧ CHAPTER 4: STRESS AND MENTAL HEALTH

Page

97. One study measured electrical activity ...: RJ Davidson and J Kabat-Zinn, 'Alterations in brain and immune function produced by mindfulness meditation', *Psychosomatic Medicine*, Jul-Aug 2003; 65 (4): pp. 64–70.

❧ CHAPTER 5: ILLICIT DRUGS

Page

104. In Australia, illicit drug use ...: Australian Institute Health and Welfare, 27 July 2011, '2010 National Drug Strategy Household Survey Report', Australian Government, http://www.aihw.gov.au/ publication-detail/?id=32212254712

105. 35.4 per cent of the Australian ...: ibid.

105. It is estimated that at least ...: ibid.

106. Hand-rolled, unfiltered marijuana ...: National Institute on Drug Abuse, 20 June 2000, 'Study Finds Marijuana Ingredient Promotes Tumor Growth, Impairs Anti-Tumor Defenses', National Institutes of Health, http://archives.drugabuse.gov/newsroom/00/NR6-20. html

107. About 10 per cent of the Australian ...: Australian Institute Health and Welfare, '2010 National Drug Strategy Household Survey Report', Australian Government.

110. It is estimated that the content ...: C Godkin, J Caulkins and P Dietze, 2005, 'Examination of heroin and amphetamine purity in

Victoria', Drug Policy Modeling Program, Bulletin 7, http://ndarc.
med.unsw.edu.au/sites/ndarc.cms.med.unsw.edu.au/files/ndarc/
resources/Bulletin%207.pdf

110. According to 2010 figures ...: Australian Institute Health and
Welfare, '2010 National Drug Strategy Household Survey Report',
Australian Government.

112. 1.4 per cent of people ...: Australian Institute Health and Welfare,
'2010 National Drug Strategy Household Survey Report', Australian
Government.

113. 46 Per cent of regular ecstasy ...: ibid.

❧ CHAPTER 7: NUTRITION

Page

133. The World Health Organization estimates ...: World Health
Organization, May 2012, 'Obesity and overweight', http://www.
who.int/mediacentre/factsheets/fs311/en/

133. There is a direct link ...: Cancer Council Victoria, 2012, 'How does
the risk vary?', http://www.cancervic.org.au/preventing-cancer/
weight/obesity-risk

133. Waist measurement has also been ...: Cancer Council Victoria,
2012, 'How does the risk vary?', www.cancervic.org.au/preventing-
cancer/weight/obesity-risk

141. A Taiwanese study found ...: RJ Yang, EK Wang, 'Irregular breakfast
eating and health status among adolescents in Taiwan', *BMC Public
Health*, 2006; 6: p. 295.

144. I want to take this opportunity ...: Q Yang, June 2012, 'Gain Weight
by "going diet"? Artificial Sweeteners and the neurobiology of sugar
cravings', *Yale Journal of Biology and Medicine*, www.ncbi.nlm.nih.
gov/pmc/articles/PMC2892765/

145. Fewer than half of Australians ...: Australian Institute of Health
and Welfare, 2012, 'Low fruit and vegetable consumption',
Australian Government, www.aihw.gov.au/risk-factors-low-fruit-
and-vegetable-consumption/

145. Regularly eating fruit reduces ...: Australian Bureau of Statistics,
2012, 'In pursuit of 2 & 5: fruit consumption in Australia', www.abs.
gov.au/ausstats/abs@.nsf/Lookup/1301.0Main+Features2362012

148. A mainly low GI diet followed ...: The Nutrition Source, 26 Nov

2012, 'Carbohydrates: good carbs guide the way', Harvard School of Public Health, www.hsph.harvard.edu/nutritionsource/what-should-you-eat/carbohydrates/index.html

152. We know from research ...: Australian Bureau of Statistics, 2012, 'In pursuit of 2 & 5: fruit and vegetable consumption in Australia', www.abs.gov.au/ausstats/abs@.nsf/Lookup/1301.0Main+Features2362012

154. If you are overweight ...: Q Yang, 'Gain Weight by "going diet?" Artificial Sweeteners and the neurobiology of sugar cravings'.

155. The sale of organic food ...: F Cottle and J Twine, 'Market Report 2012', Soil Association, www.soilassociation.org/marketreport

155. The most often-cited ...: PRD Williams and JK Hammitt, 2001, 'Perceived Risks of Conventional and organic Produce: pesticides, pathogens and Natural Toxins', *Risk Analysis*, vol. 21, no. 2. http://expeng.anr.msu.edu/uploads/files/31/perceived%20risks%20with%20conv%20vs%20organic.pdf

156. In recent US studies ...: C Lu et al., 'Organic diets significantly lower children's dietary exposure to organophosphorus pesticides', *Environmental Health Perspectives*, February 2006; 114 (2): pp. 260–3. Source: Department of Environmental and Occupational Health, Rollins School of Public Health, Emory University, Atlanta, Georgia, USA.

156. We know that pesticide ...: ibid.

162. This fact was recognised ...: National Health and Medical Research Council, 12 October 2012, Dietary Guidelines for all Australians, Australian Government, www.nhmrc.gov.au/guidelines/publications/n29-n30-n31-n32-n33-n34

❧ CHAPTER 9: EXERCISE

Page

174. A compelling argument ...: R Ballard-Barbash et al., Physical Activity Linked To Reduced Mortality in Breast and Colon Cancer Patients', *JNCI Journal National Cancer Institute*, 8 May 2012, 104(11).

174. Competitive sport in childhood ...: M Nilsson and C Ohlsson et al., 'Competitive physical activity early in life is associated with bone mineral density in elderly Swedish men.' *Osteoporosis International*, 2008; 19(11):1557–1566.

175. Swimming, however ...: JW Bellew and L Gehrig, 'A comparison of bone mineral density in adolescent female swimmers, soccer players, and weight lifters.' *Pediatric Physical Therapy*, 2006; 18(1): pp. 19–22.

175. Research studies have shown ...: D Nieman, 'Regular Moderate Exercise boosts immunity', *AgroFOOD*, May/June 2008, vol. 19, no. 3, http://chemistry-today.teknoscienze.com/pdf/NIEMAN%20 AGRO3-08.pdf

176. Think you're too old ...: RS Paffenbarger Jr, RT Hyde, AL Wing, CC Hsieh, 'Physical activity, all-cause mortality, and longevity of college alumni', *The New England Journal of Medicine*, 1986; 314: pp. 605–13.

176. Rate of sedentary and low ...: World Health Organisation, 2012, 'Global Strategy on Diet, Physical Activity, and Health', www.who. int/dietphysicalactivity/childhood_why/en/index.html

176. Females (73 per cent) ...: ibid.

176. Over 75 years of age ...: ibid.

176. The rate is lowest ...: ibid.

176. Children are more likely ...: ibid.

176. Internationally, the data ...: ibid.

176. Physical activity levels ...: ibid.

🌿 CHAPTER 10: IMMUNITY

Page

189. There is strong evidence ...: JM Mullington et al., 'Cardiovascular, Inflammatory and Metabolic Consequences of Sleep Deprivation' *Progress in Cardiovascular Disease*, 2009 Jan-Feb; 51(4): 294–302.

189. We know that excess fat ...: J Lysaght, 'Pro-inflammatory and tumour proliferative properties of excess visceral adipose tissue', *Cancer Letters*, Dec 2011, 15;312(1):62–72. Epub 2011 Aug 11.

189. Type 2 diabetes and insulin resistance: DJ Rader, 'Effect of insulin resistance, dyslipidemia, and intra-abdominal adiposity on the development of cardiovascular disease and diabetes mellitus', *American Journal Medicine*, 2007 Mar;120(3 Suppl 1):S12–8.

189. Sleep disruption reduces ...: NL Rogers et al., 'Neuroimmunologic aspects of sleep and sleep loss', *Seminars in Clinical Neuropsychiatry*, 2001, 6(4): pp. 295–307.

Page

193. People with cancer who ...: C Puchalski, 'The Role of Spirituality in health care', *Proceedings* (Baylor University Medical Centre), 2001 October; 14(4): pp. 352–357.

194. Some of the known health benefits ...: K Phelps and C Hassed, *General Practice: the Integrative Approach*, Elsevier 2010.

195. Medical research has turned ...: ibid.

195. Spirituality has been shown ...: B Doolittle, 'The Association Between Spirituality and Depression in an Urban Clinic Prim Care Companion', *Journal of Clinical Psychiatry*, 2004; 6 (3): pp. 114–8. PMCID: PMC474734.

196. People undergoing heart surgery ...: T Oxman, D Freeman, E Manheimer, 'Lack of social participation or religious strength and comfort as risk factors for death after cardiac surgery in the elderly', *Psychosomatic Medicine*, 1995; 57: pp. 5–15.

199. The opposite of connectedness ...: JT Cacciopo and LC Hawkley, 'Social isolation and health, with an emphasis on underlying mechanisms', *Perspectives in Biology and Medicine*, 2003 Summer; 46(3 Suppl):S39–52.

199. Substance abuse and domestic violence: KL Chou et al., 'The association between social isolation and DSM-IV mood, anxiety, and substance use disorders: wave 2 of the National Epidemiologic Survey on Alcohol and Related Conditions', *Journal of Clinical Psychiatry*, 2011 Nov;72(11):1468–76. Epub 2011 Jan 11.

201. Research has shown us ...: K Orth-Gomér, SP Wamala, M Horsten et al., 'Marital stress worsens prognosis in women with coronary heart disease: the Stockholm Female Coronary Risk Study', *Cardiovascular Quality and Outcomes*, JAMA 2000; 284:3008–3014.

201. A recent meta-analysis ...: J Holt-Lunstad, TB Smith, JB Layton, 'Social relationships and mortality risk: A meta-analytic review', *Public Library of Science Medicine*, 2010; 7: e1000316. doi: 10.1371/journal.pmed.1000316.

201. Social support in the form of marriage ...: DH Jaffe, O Manor, Z Eisenbach et al., 'The protective effect of marriage on mortality in a dynamic society', *Annals of Epidemiology*, 2007; 17(7): pp. 540–547.

209. By age 65 ...: National Institute Deafness and Other Communication Disorders, October 1997, 'Presbycusis', National Institute of Health, www.nidcd.nih.gov/health/hearing/pages/presbycusis.aspx

213. Studies have shown ...: PW Lin et al., 'Efficacy of aromatherapy (Lavandula angustifolia) as an intervention for agitated behaviours in Chinese older persons with dementia: a cross-over randomized trial', *International Journal of Geriatric Psychiatry*, 2007 May;22(5): pp. 405–10.

214. 'dry, full of extremes ...': Australian Government, 'Australian Humour', http://australia.gov.au/about-australia/australian-story/austn-humour

SECTION 4 INTEGRATED MEDICINE AND COMPLEMENTARY TREATMENTS

❧ CHAPTER 1: ACUPUNCTURE AND PHYSICAL THERAPIES

Page

221. They found that there was evidence ...: National Institutes of Health, 5 November 1997, 'NIH Panel Issue Consensus Statement on Acupuncture', http://www.nih.gov/news/pr/nov97/od-05.htm

❧ CHAPTER 2: TAKING THE RIGHT PHARMACEUTICAL DRUGS

Page

229. Studies have shown that ...: L Roughead and S Semple, July 2002, 'Second National Report on Patient Safety - Improving Medication Safety', Australian Council for Safety and Quality in Health Care, http://www.safetyandquality.gov.au/wp-content/uploads/2012/01/med_saf_rept.pdf

230. Each year in Australia ...: E Roughhead and J Lexchin, 'Adverse drug events: counting is not enough, action is needed', *Medical Journal of Australia*, vol.184, no. 7, 3 April 2006.

230. Based on an estimate ...: ibid.

230. These ADEs are not trivial ...: ibid.

🌿 CHAPTER 3: HERBAL MEDICINE

Page

246. And larger studies ...: ST De Kosky et al., '*Ginkgo biloba* for Prevention of Dementia: A Randomized Controlled Trial', *The Journal of American Medicine Association*, 2008;300(19):2253–2262. doi:10.1001/jama.2008.683.

STEP 3: SUSTAIN

🌿 YOUR NEW NORMAL

Page

291. After studying the social connections and body ...: NA Christakis and JH Fowler, 'The Spread of Obesity in a Large Social Network Over 32 Years', *New England Journal of Medicine*, 2007; 357: pp. 370–379.

INDEX

cancer
  exercise and 174
  toxins and 54
cannabis 105–7
  active ingredients 105
  long-term effects 106
  quitting 106–7
  short-term effects 105–6
carbohydrates 147–8
  GI (glycaemic index) 148
cardiovascular disease
  exercise and protection from 173–4
cardiovascular fitness 2
chamomile tea 126
chaste tree (*Vitex agnus castus*) 241–2
chelation therapy 63
chiropractic therapy 39, 224
chiropractor 45–6
chlorella 62
chlorophyll 62
chromium 268–9
cigarettes *see* smoking
cocaine 110–12
  long-term effects 111–12
  short-term effects 111
  use in Australia 110
coenzyme Q10 269
cognitive behaviour therapy (CBT) 100, 123
complementary and alternative medicine (CAM) 5, 7–8, 218
  acceptance by doctors 39
  definition 7
  herbal *see* herbal medicine
  poor use of 10
  rates of practice and referral by Australian GPs 38
  Traditional Chinese Medicine (TCM) *see* Traditional Chinese Medicine practitioners/techniques
connectedness 193, 196–205
  audit 199–200
  circles of 197–8
  goals 216–17
connection
  damaging relationships 201–2
  finding your 'tribe' 200–1
  forgiveness 202–3
  friendships 205
  home life 205

hostility, eliminating 202
  making new connections 204–5
  other people, with 196–205
  reaching out 203–5
  senses, with 206–13 *see also* senses
  social isolation 199
  social media, through 198–9
  3 am people 197
Consumer Medicines Information leaflets 13
counselling 123
counsellor 47–8
cramps, abdominal 31
cranberry (*Vaccinium macrocarpum*) 242
cyanocobalamin 262–3

dairy products 146
deafness 209
delirium tremens (DTs) 76
dental check-ups 19
depression 85
  medications causing 102
  stress and 101–2
detox 51–65
  aim 51
  alcohol 59–60, 74–5
  caffeine 59
  diet 58–9
  duration 63–4
  elimination process 56–7
  exercise 62
  health problems related to toxin exposure/overload 53–5
  heavy metals 63
  identification of toxins 55–6
  illicit drugs 60
  mercury fillings 60–1
  mind, of 62–3
  phases 64–5
  prerequisite 54
  process 51, 55–65
  restoring balance 64
  sleep 62
  stress, reduction of 62–3
  supplements to support 61–2
  toxin audit, use of 55, 57
  toxins in body 52–3
  volatile organic compounds (VOCs) 57–8
  what is 51